The Autoimmune Protocol Diet Cookbook for Beginners

2000 Days of Delicious and Nourishing AIP Paleo Recipes to Help You Reverse Autoimmune Diseases, Boost Immune System Function, and Heal Your Thyroid through the 4 Dietary Stages.

Eugene M. Howard

Table of Contents

Introduction: Welcome to the AIP Journey!

Welcome to *"The Autoimmune Protocol Diet Cookbook for Beginners,"* your comprehensive guide to embracing the Autoimmune Protocol (AIP) diet. This journey goes beyond food; it's about reclaiming your health, recognizing your body's needs, and discovering the profound link between your diet and health. The AIP diet aims to manage autoimmune disorders by reducing inflammation, healing the digestive tract, and identifying food sensitivities. As you progress on this journey, you will discover that the AIP diet is not all about restrictions alone but rather a pathway to nourishment and wellness.

Understanding the Role of Diet in Autoimmune Health

Diet is critical for treating autoimmune diseases. Autoimmune disorders occur when the immune system mistakenly assaults its own tissues, resulting in chronic inflammation and various health problems. Foods can either worsen or help alleviate inflammation. The AIP diet emphasizes nutrient-dense, anti-inflammatory foods while avoiding possible triggers such as grains, dairy, and processed foods. The AIP diet, which prioritizes vegetables, lean meats, healthy fats, and gut-healing foods, attempts to restore immune system balance and improve overall wellness. Understanding this relationship allows you to make informed choices that benefit your health and vitality.

How To Use This Cookbook

"The Autoimmune Protocol Diet Cookbook for Beginners" is designed to help you navigate every stage of your AIP journey. Whether you're new to the AIP diet or seeking new inspiration, this cookbook has numerous delicious and nutrient-dense recipes tailored to your specific needs. Each section provides:

- **Clear Guidelines:** Know the AIP diet principles and how to apply them to your daily routine.
- **Easy-to-Follow Recipes:** Step-by-step directions for cooking delectable, AIP-compliant meals.
- **Meal Planning Tips:** Organize your shopping, cooking, and meal prep to make the AIP diet more manageable and pleasurable.
- **Reintroduction Guidance:** Learn how to systematically reintroduce foods and discover personal triggers while expanding your diet.

Use this cookbook as a companion and reference guide. Explore new ingredients, enjoy the flavors of therapeutic foods, and feel empowered knowing you're taking proactive measures toward better health. Enjoy the journey, and let each recipe be a step toward achieving optimal wellness.

Chapter 1

Understanding Autoimmune Diseases

Overview of Autoimmune Diseases

Autoimmune diseases develop when the body's immune system, which typically defends it against hazardous intruders such as germs and viruses, mistakenly attacks its own tissues. This misdirected immune response causes chronic inflammation and damage to many organs and systems. There are over 80 forms of autoimmune disorders, each affecting a distinct portion of the body. Common autoimmune disorders include:

- Rheumatoid arthritis, which affects the joints.

- Lupus, which affects the skin, kidneys, and other organs.

- Multiple sclerosis, which affects the nervous system.

- Hashimoto's thyroiditis, which affects the thyroid gland.

Understanding autoimmune disorders is the first step toward managing and reducing their effects on health.

Causes and Risk Factors

Although the causes of autoimmune diseases are not fully understood, a combination of genetic, environmental, and lifestyle factors is believed to contribute to their development.

- **Genetic Factors:** A family history of autoimmune diseases can raise your risk. Certain genes have been found to increase the likelihood of developing autoimmunity, but it's important to note that having these genes doesn't necessarily mean that the disease will develop.
- **Environmental Factors:** Exposure to some environmental triggers, such as infections, toxins, and even certain foods, can activate the immune system in ways that promote autoimmunity. Stress and trauma also play a significant role.
- **Lifestyle Factors:** The risk and severity of autoimmune diseases can be influenced by factors such as diet, physical activity, and overall lifestyle. A diet primarily consisting of processed foods and lacking essential nutrients can exacerbate inflammation. Smoking and lack of exercise are also contributing factors.

By recognizing these factors, you can make informed choices to decrease their risk and better manage existing conditions.

Symptoms and Diagnosis

The symptoms of autoimmune diseases can vary greatly depending on the specific condition and the organs affected. However, there are typical symptoms that many autoimmune diseases have in common, including:

- Chronic fatigue

- Pain and swelling in the joints
- Muscle aches
- Skin rashes
- Digestive problems
- Recurring fevers
- Swollen lymph nodes

Diagnosing autoimmune diseases can be quite challenging because of the overlapping nature of symptoms and their variability. Healthcare professionals employ a variety of techniques to diagnose these conditions accurately:

- **Medical History and Physical Exam:** A comprehensive assessment of symptoms and family history, combined with a physical examination, can offer valuable initial insights.
- **Blood Tests:** Certain antibodies and markers of inflammation in the blood can provide valuable insights into the presence of an autoimmune process. Typical tests include ANA (antinuclear antibody), CRP (C-reactive protein), and ESR (erythrocyte sedimentation rate).
- **Imaging and Biopsies:** Imaging techniques such as X-rays, MRIs, and ultrasounds effectively detect internal inflammation and damage. In certain situations, a biopsy of the affected tissue may be required to establish a conclusive diagnosis.

Early and accurate diagnosis is essential for successful management and treatment. Having an excellent grasp of the symptoms and diagnostic process allows individuals to promptly seek medical advice and start appropriate interventions to manage their autoimmune conditions.

Chapter 2

The Autoimmune Protocol (AIP) Diet

A Brief Overview of the AIP Diet

The Autoimmune Protocol (AIP) diet is a specialized diet focusing on reducing inflammation, promoting gut health, and managing autoimmune conditions. This diet is an extension of the Paleo diet, with a focus on nutrient-dense, whole foods. It also eliminates potential dietary triggers that may cause immune system reactions. The principles behind the AIP diet involve:

- Eliminating foods that cause inflammation.

- Promoting gut healing.

- Identifying food sensitivities through a structured reintroduction phase.

By following the AIP diet, individuals frequently notice decreased symptoms, increased energy levels, and enhanced overall health.

Foods to Avoid and Include

Foods to avoid

The AIP diet focuses on eliminating foods that can trigger inflammation and worsen symptoms of autoimmune conditions. Here are some examples:

- Grains such as wheat, rice, oats, etc.
- Dairy products
- Legumes (beans, lentils, and peanuts).
- Vegetables like tomatoes, potatoes, eggplants, and peppers
- Eggs
- Assorted nuts and seeds
- Processed foods and food additives
- Refined sugars and sweeteners
- Alcohol and caffeine

Foods to Include

On the other hand, the AIP diet promotes the intake of wholesome and nutritious foods that help boost immune function and maintain gut health. Here are some examples:

- Vegetables (excluding nightshades)
- Fruits (in moderation).
- High-quality meats and organ meats
- Seafood
- Healthy fats (olive oil, coconut oil, avocado oil)
- Fermented foods (sauerkraut, kimchi, and kombucha)

- Bone broth
- Herbs and spices (excluding nightshade spices like paprika and cayenne)

Nutritional Guidelines

Maintaining a well-rounded nutrient intake is vital when adhering to the AIP diet. Here are some helpful suggestions for maintaining proper nutrition:

- **Variety:** Include a wide selection of vegetables, fruits, and protein sources to guarantee a broad spectrum of vitamins and minerals.
- **Healthy Fats:** Incorporate healthy fats into your diet by including sources of omega-3 fatty acids like fatty fish, flaxseed oil, and chia seeds. These can help reduce inflammation.
- **Bone Health:** Ensure strong bones by incorporating bone broth and leafy green vegetables into your diet to boost calcium intake.
- **Improve Gut Health:** Incorporate fermented foods and probiotics into your diet to support a healthy gut microbiome.
- **Hydration:** Drink plenty of water throughout the day to stay hydrated and support overall health.
- **Moderation:** Although fruits are allowed, consume them in moderation to avoid excessive sugar intake.

Tips for Shopping and Essential Pantry Items

To successfully follow the AIP diet, it's essential to stock your kitchen with AIP-friendly ingredients and plan your shopping trips effectively:

Helpful Shopping Tips

- **Be Prepared:** Create a meal plan and shopping list in advance so you can easily get all the ingredients you need when you visit the store.
- **Examine Labels:** Read ingredient lists to uncover any hidden additives, sugars, or nightshade spices that are not AIP-compliant.
- **Prioritize Freshness:** Prioritize fresh, whole foods from the produce and meat sections.
- Frozen Options: It's a good idea to keep frozen vegetables and fruits on hand for convenience and ensure you always have AIP-friendly options.
- **Bulk Buying:** Save money and reduce the frequency of shopping trips by purchasing items like coconut oil, olive oil, and frozen meats in bulk.

Essential Items for Your Pantry

Make meal preparation easier by stocking your pantry with these essential items for the AIP diet:

- **Oils:** Olive oil, coconut oil, and avocado oil
- **Flours:** Coconut flour, arrowroot flour, tapioca flour
- **Broth:** Bone broth (homemade or store-bought with high-quality ingredients)
- **Spices:** Turmeric, ginger, garlic powder, cinnamon, and other non-nightshade spices
- **Canned Goods:** Wild-caught fish and coconut milk without any additives.
- **Fermented Foods:** Sauerkraut, kimchi, kombucha
- **Snacks:** Dried fruits (without added sugar), plantain chips, coconut flakes

By following these guidelines and tips, you can create a supportive environment that makes sticking to the AIP diet easier.

Chapter 3

60-Day AIP Meal Plan for the Four Stages

2-Week Elimination Phase Meal Plan

Day	Breakfast	Lunch	Dinner	Snacks
1	Sweet Potato Hash with Sausage and Spinach (Page 13)	Zucchini Noodles with Ground Turkey and Avocado Pesto (Page 25)	Baked Salmon with Asparagus and Mashed Cauliflower (Page 37)	Apple Slices with Coconut Butter (Page 49)
2	Zucchini and Bacon Fritters (Page 14)	Chicken and Vegetable Soup (Page 26)	Braised Lamb Shanks with Root Vegetables (Page 38)	Plantain Chips with Guacamole (Page 50)
3	Apple-Cinnamon Cauliflower Porridge (Page 15)	Tuna Salad Lettuce Wraps (Page 27)	AIP Meatloaf with Sweet Potato Mash (Page 39)	Carrot and Celery Sticks with AIP Ranch Dip (Page 51)
4	Breakfast Sausage Patties with Sautéed Greens (Page 16)	Shrimp and Mango Salad (Page 28)	Coconut-Crusted Cod with Steamed Broccoli (Page 40)	AIP Beef Jerky (Page 52)
5	Coconut Yogurt with Blueberries and Honey (Page 17)	Beef and Broccoli Stir-fry (Page 29)	Herb-Roasted Chicken with Brussels Sprouts (Page 41)	Mixed Berry Fruit Leather (Page 53)
6	AIP Pumpkin Pancakes with Maple Syrup (Page 18)	AIP Caesar Salad with Grilled Chicken (Page 30)	Beef and Vegetable Stew (Page 42)	Coconut Macaroons (Page 54)
7	Banana and Coconut Smoothie (Page 19)	Turkey and Apple Slaw (Page 31)	Lemon-Garlic Shrimp with Zucchini Noodles (Page 43)	Baked Kale Chips (Page 55)
8	Carrot and Parsnip Hash Browns (Page 20)	Salmon Salad with Cucumber and Dill (Page 32)	Pork Tenderloin with Apple Compote (Page 44)	Avocado and Tuna Boats (Page 56)
9	Smoked Salmon and Avocado Salad (Page 21)	AIP Cobb Salad with Balsamic Dressing (Page 33)	Ginger-Turmeric Chicken Thighs with Cauliflower Rice (Page 45)	AIP Granola Bars with Coconut and Dried Fruit (Page 57)
10	Cauliflower Rice Breakfast Bowl (Page 22)	Grilled Chicken with Mixed Greens and Lemon Vinaigrette (Page 34)	AIP Shepherd's Pie with Ground Beef and Carrot Mash (Page 46)	Cucumber Slices with Smoked Salmon (Page 58)
11	Chicken Apple Breakfast Meatballs (Page 23)	AIP BLT Salad with Avocado Dressing (Page 35)	Coconut Chicken Curry with Cauliflower Rice (Page 47)	Mango and Pineapple Smoothie (Page 59)

12	Butternut Squash and Sage Breakfast Skillet (Page 24)	Roasted Vegetable and Herb Salad (Page 36)	Grilled Steak with Sautéed Spinach and Garlic (Page 48)	Coconut Milk Popsicles with Berries (Page 60)
13	Sweet Potato Hash with Sausage and Spinach (Page 13)	Zucchini Noodles with Ground Turkey and Avocado Pesto (Page 25)	Baked Salmon with Asparagus and Mashed Cauliflower (Page 37)	Apple Slices with Coconut Butter (Page 49)
14	Zucchini and Bacon Fritters (Page 14)	Chicken and Vegetable Soup (Page 26)	Braised Lamb Shanks with Root Vegetables (Page 38)	Plantain Chips with Guacamole (Page 50)

2-Week Maintenance Phase Meal Plan

Day	Breakfast	Lunch	Dinner	Snacks
1	Sweet Potato and Kale Breakfast Hash (Page 62)	Grilled Chicken Salad with Mixed Greens and Avocado (Page 74)	Herb-Roasted Chicken with Brussels Sprouts (Page 86)	Apple Slices with Almond Butter (Page 98)
2	Zucchini and Bacon Fritters with Avocado (Page 63)	Turkey and Cranberry Lettuce Wraps (Page 75)	Baked Salmon with Asparagus and Lemon Dill Sauce (Page 87)	Carrot and Celery Sticks with AIP Ranch Dip (Page 99)
3	Coconut Yogurt Parfait with Berries and Honey (Page 64)	Shrimp and Mango Salad with Lime Vinaigrette (Page 76)	Beef and Vegetable Stew with Sweet Potatoes (Page 88)	Homemade AIP Granola Bars with Pumpkin Seeds (Page 100)
4	Scrambled Eggs with Spinach and Mushrooms (Page 65)	Beef and Broccoli Stir-fry with Coconut Aminos (Page 77)	Pork Tenderloin with Apple Compote and Roasted Carrots (Page 89)	Baked Kale Chips with Sea Salt (Page 101)
5	Banana and Flaxseed Smoothie (Page 66)	AIP Caesar Salad with Homemade Dressing and Anchovies (Page 78)	Lemon-Garlic Shrimp with Zucchini Noodles (Page 90)	Coconut Macaroons with Dark Chocolate Drizzle (Page 102)
6	Chia Seed Pudding with Mango and Coconut (Page 67)	Tuna Salad with Cucumber and Dill (Page 79)	Lamb Chops with Mint and Roasted Root Vegetables (Page 91)	Deviled Eggs with Avocado and Paprika (Page 103)
7	AIP Pancakes with Maple Syrup and Blueberries (Page 68)	Roasted Vegetable and Herb Salad with Chicken (Page 80)	Grilled Steak with Chimichurri Sauce and Cauliflower Rice (Page 92)	Mixed Berry Fruit Leather (Page 104)

8	Breakfast Sausage Patties with Sweet Potato Mash (Page 69)	Mixed Greens Salad with Egg Yolks and Olive Oil Dressing (Page 81)	Coconut Chicken Curry with Cauliflower Rice (Page 93)	Plantain Chips with Guacamole (Page 105)
9	Avocado Toast on AIP Bread with Poached Eggs (Page 70)	Grilled Salmon with Arugula and Pomegranate Seeds (Page 82)	AIP Meatloaf with Mashed Parsnips (Page 94)	AIP Beef Jerky with Herbs (Page 106)
10	Mixed Berry Smoothie Bowl with Hemp Seeds (Page 71)	Turkey and Apple Slaw with Carrot-Ginger Dressing (Page 83)	Ginger-Turmeric Chicken Thighs with Broccoli (Page 95)	Chia Seed Pudding with Coconut Milk and Honey (Page 107)
11	Butternut Squash and Apple Hash (Page 72)	Zucchini Noodles with Walnut Pesto and Cherry Tomatoes (Page 84)	Baked Cod with Almond Crust and Green Beans (Page 96)	Sliced Cucumbers with Smoked Salmon and Dill (Page 108)
12	Smoked Salmon and Dill Omelette (Page 73)	Baked Cod with Spinach and Avocado Salsa (Page 85)	Stuffed Bell Peppers with Ground Beef and Vegetables (Page 97)	Trail Mix with Nuts and Dried Fruit (Page 109)
13	Sweet Potato and Kale Breakfast Hash (Page 62)	Grilled Chicken Salad with Mixed Greens and Avocado (Page 74)	Herb-Roasted Chicken with Brussels Sprouts (Page 86)	Apple Slices with Almond Butter (Page 98)
14	Zucchini and Bacon Fritters with Avocado (Page 63)	Turkey and Cranberry Lettuce Wraps (Page 75)	Baked Salmon with Asparagus and Lemon Dill Sauce (Page 87)	Carrot and Celery Sticks with AIP Ranch Dip (Page 99)

2-Week Personalization Phase Meal Plan

Day	Breakfast	Lunch	Dinner	Snacks
1	Sweet Potato and Spinach Breakfast Hash (Page 111)	Grilled Chicken Salad with Mixed Greens and Citrus Vinaigrette (Page 123)	Herb-Roasted Chicken with Brussels Sprouts and Sweet Potato Mash (Page 136)	Apple Slices with Almond Butter and Cinnamon (Page 148)
2	Coconut Yogurt Parfait with Mixed Berries and Flax Seeds (Page 112)	Turkey and Cranberry Lettuce Wraps with Pumpkin Seeds Vinaigrette (Page 125)	Baked Salmon with Asparagus and Lemon Dill Sauce Potato Mash (Page 137)	Carrot and Celery Sticks with AIP Ranch Dip (Page 149)
3	Scrambled Eggs with Sautéed Mushrooms and Kale (Page 113)	Shrimp and Avocado Salad with Lime Dressing (Page 126)	Beef and Vegetable Stew with Root Vegetables Mash (Page 138)	Homemade AIP Granola Bars with Pumpkin Seeds and Coconut (Page 150)
4	Banana and Almond Butter Smoothie (Page 114)	Beef and Broccoli Stir-fry with Coconut Aminos and Cashews (Page 127)	Pork Tenderloin with Apple Compote and Roasted Carrots (Page 139)	Baked Kale Chips with Sea Salt and Olive Oil (Page 151)
5	Chia Seed Pudding with Mango and Blueberries (Page 115)	AIP Caesar Salad with Homemade Dressing and Sardines (Page 128)	Lemon-Garlic Shrimp with Zucchini Noodles and Pesto (Page 140)	Coconut Macaroons with Dark Chocolate Drizzle (Page 152)
6	Cassava Flour Pancakes with Maple Syrup and Strawberries (Page 116)	Tuna Salad with Cucumber, Dill, and Lemon (Page 129)	Lamb Chops with Mint, Roasted Root Vegetables, and Pomegranate Seeds (Page 141)	Deviled Eggs with Avocado and Smoked Paprika (Page 153)
7	Breakfast Sausage Patties with Apple Slices (Page 117)	Roasted Vegetable and Quinoa Salad with Chicken (Page 130)	Grilled Steak with Chimichurri Sauce and Cauliflower Rice (Page 142)	Mixed Berry Fruit Leather with Honey (Page 154)
8	Avocado Toast on AIP Bread with Soft-Boiled Eggs (Page 118)	Mixed Greens Salad with Egg Yolks and Olive Oil Dressing (Page 131)	Coconut Chicken Curry with Cauliflower Rice and Spinach (Page 143)	Plantain Chips with Guacamole and Salsa (Page 155)
9	Green Smoothie Bowl with Hemp Seeds and Kiwi (Page 119)	Grilled Salmon with Arugula, Pomegranate Seeds, and Almonds (Page 132)	AIP Meatloaf with Mashed Parsnips and Green Beans (Page 144)	AIP Beef Jerky with Herbs and Garlic (Page 156)
10	Butternut Squash and Apple Breakfast Bake (Page 120)	Turkey and Apple Slaw with Carrot-Ginger Dressing (Page 133)	Ginger-Turmeric Chicken Thighs with Roasted Broccoli (Page 145)	Chia Seed Pudding with Coconut Milk, Honey, and

				Blueberries (Page 157)
11	Smoked Salmon and Cucumber Salad (Page 121)	Zucchini Noodles with Walnut Pesto and Cherry Tomatoes (Page 134)	Baked Cod with Almond Crust, Green Beans, and Carrot Purée (Page 146)	Sliced Cucumbers with Smoked Salmon and Dill (Page 158)
12	Zucchini Noodles with Poached Eggs and Avocado (Page 122)	Baked Cod with Spinach, Avocado Salsa, and Sweet Potatoes (Page 135)	Stuffed Bell Peppers with Ground Beef, Quinoa, and Spinach (Page 147)	Trail Mix with Nuts, Seeds, and Dried Fruit (Page 159)
13	Sweet Potato and Spinach Breakfast Hash (Page 111)	Grilled Chicken Salad with Mixed Greens and Citrus Vinaigrette (Page 123)	Herb-Roasted Chicken with Brussels Sprouts and Sweet Potato Mash (Page 136)	Apple Slices with Almond Butter and Cinnamon (Page 148)
14	Coconut Yogurt Parfait with Mixed Berries and Flax Seeds (Page 112)	Turkey and Cranberry Lettuce Wraps with Pumpkin Seeds Vinaigrette (Page 125)	Baked Salmon with Asparagus and Lemon Dill Sauce Potato Mash (Page 137)	Carrot and Celery Sticks with AIP Ranch Dip (Page 149)

2-Week Reintroduction Phase Meal Plan

Day	Breakfast	Lunch	Dinner	Snacks
1	Spinach and Egg Yolk Salad with Lemon Dressing (Page 161)	Grilled Chicken Salad with Sesame Dressing (Page 172)	Tomato-Basil Chicken with Roasted Sweet Potatoes (Page 183)	Deviled Eggs with Avocado (Page 195)
2	Banana Pancakes with Almond Butter (Page 162)	Turkey Wraps with Almond Flour Tortillas (Page 173)	Grilled Steak with Chimichurri Sauce (Page 184)	Apple Slices with Almond Butter (Page 196)
3	Sweet Potato Hash with Cashew Cream (Page 163)	Mixed Greens Salad with Egg Yolk Vinaigrette (Page 174)	Pork Tenderloin with Apple and Walnut Stuffing (Page 185)	Chia Seed Pudding with Coconut Milk and Honey (Page 197)
4	Chia Seed Pudding with Berries (Page 164)	Beef Stir-fry with Bell Peppers (Page 175)	Lemon-Garlic Shrimp with Spaghetti Squash and Pesto (Page 186)	Celery Sticks with Sunflower Seed Butter (Page 198)
5	Scrambled Eggs with Avocado and Salsa (Page 165)	Salmon Salad with Avocado and Flaxseed Oil (Page 176)	Beef and Vegetable Skewers with Bell Peppers (Page 187)	Trail Mix with Nuts and Dried Fruit (Page 199)
6	Breakfast Smoothie with Flax Seeds (Page 166)	Zucchini Noodles with Walnut Pesto (Page 177)	Herb-Crusted Salmon with Flaxseed Crust (Page 188)	Baked Plantain Chips with

				Guacamole (Page 200)
7	Egg Muffins with Spinach and Mushrooms (Page 167)	Chicken Caesar Salad with Egg Yolks in Dressing (Page 178)	Chicken Alfredo with Cashew Cream Sauce (Page 189)	AIP Energy Balls with Flaxseeds (Page 201)
8	Butternut Squash Breakfast Bowl with Pumpkin Seeds (Page 168)	AIP BLT Salad with Avocado and Tomato (Page 179)	AIP Meatloaf with Egg Yolks (Page 190)	Homemade Granola Bars with Pumpkin Seeds (Page 202)
9	Avocado Toast on AIP Bread with Egg Yolk (Page 169)	Shrimp and Mango Salad with Sesame Seeds (Page 180)	Lamb Chops with Mint and Pomegranate Salad (Page 191)	Mixed Berry Smoothie with Almond Milk (Page 203)
10	Mixed Berry Smoothie with Hemp Seeds (Page 170)	Turkey and Cranberry Salad with Pecans (Page 181)	Stuffed Bell Peppers with Ground Beef and Vegetables (Page 192)	Raw Veggies with Tahini Dip (Page 204)
11	AIP Breakfast Sausage with Poached Eggs (Page 171)	Spinach and Mushroom Salad with Poached Eggs (Page 182)	Baked Cod with Almond Crust (Page 193)	Coconut Macaroons with Egg Whites (Page 205)
12	Spinach and Egg Yolk Salad with Lemon Dressing (Page 161)	Grilled Chicken Salad with Sesame Dressing (Page 172)	Ginger-Turmeric Chicken Thighs with Tomato Relish (Page 194)	Sliced Cucumbers with Smoked Salmon and Dill (Page 206)
13	Banana Pancakes with Almond Butter (Page 162)	Turkey Wraps with Almond Flour Tortillas (Page 173)	Tomato-Basil Chicken with Roasted Sweet Potatoes (Page 183)	Deviled Eggs with Avocado (Page 195)
14	Sweet Potato Hash with Cashew Cream (Page 163)	Mixed Greens Salad with Egg Yolk Vinaigrette (Page 174)	Grilled Steak with Chimichurri Sauce (Page 184)	Apple Slices with Almond Butter (Page 196)

Chapter 4: Elimination Phase Recipes

Breakfast Recipes

Sweet Potato Hash with Sausage and Spinach

Prep Time: 15 minutes | **Cook Time:** 25 minutes | **Servings:** 4

Ingredients:

- 2 large sweet potatoes, peeled and diced
- 1-pound ground pork sausage (AIP-compliant, no additives)
- 1 medium onion, diced
- 2 cloves garlic, minced
- 2 cups fresh spinach, chopped
- 2 tablespoons coconut oil
- 1 teaspoon sea salt
- 1 teaspoon dried thyme
- 1 teaspoon dried rosemary
- 1/2 teaspoon ground turmeric
- 1/4 teaspoon ground ginger

Instructions:

1. Heat 1 tablespoon of coconut oil in a large skillet over medium heat. Add the diced onion and minced garlic, cooking until the onion is translucent.

2. Add the ground pork sausage to the skillet. Cook, breaking it up with a spoon, until it is browned and fully cooked.

3. Take out the sausage from the skillet and set it aside. Add the remaining 1 tablespoon of coconut oil to the skillet.

4. Add the diced sweet potatoes to the skillet. Cook, stirring occasionally, until they are tender and starting to brown, about 10-15 minutes.

5. Return the cooked sausage to the skillet with the sweet potatoes. Add the chopped spinach, sea salt, dried thyme, dried rosemary, ground turmeric, and ground ginger. Stir to combine and cook until the spinach is wilted.

6. Serve hot.

Nutritional Information (per serving):

- **Calories:** 340 kcal
- **Fat:** 15 g
- **Carbohydrates:** 28 g
- **Proteins:** 18 g

Zucchini and Bacon Fritters

Prep Time: 20 minutes | **Cook Time:** 15 minutes | **Servings:** 4

Ingredients:

- 2 medium zucchinis, grated
- 1/2 teaspoon sea salt
- 6 slices bacon, chopped
- 1/4 cup coconut flour
- 2 tablespoons arrowroot flour
- 2 green onions, finely chopped

- 1 clove garlic, minced
- 1/2 teaspoon dried oregano
- 1/2 teaspoon dried basil
- 1/4 teaspoon ground turmeric
- 2 tablespoons coconut oil

Instructions:

1. Place the grated zucchini in a colander, sprinkle with sea salt, and let it sit for 10 minutes to draw out excess moisture. After 10 minutes, squeeze out the moisture using a clean kitchen towel or paper towels.

2. In a large skillet, cook the chopped bacon over medium heat until crispy. Take out the bacon and set it aside, leaving the bacon fat in the skillet.

3. In a large bowl, combine the squeezed zucchini, cooked bacon, coconut flour, arrowroot flour, finely chopped green onions, minced garlic, dried oregano, dried basil, and ground turmeric. Mix adequately to combine.

4. Heat the coconut oil in the same skillet over medium heat.

5. Scoop about 1/4 cup of the mixture into the skillet, flattening it slightly to form a fritter. Repeat with the remaining mixture, cooking the fritters in batches.

6. Cook each fritter for about 3-4 minutes per side, until golden brown and cooked through.

7. Take out the fritters from the skillet and place them on a paper towel-lined plate to drain any excess oil.

8. Serve hot.

Nutritional Information (per serving):

- **Calories:** 230 kcal
- **Fat:** 18 g
- **Carbohydrates:** 8 g
- **Proteins:** 10 g

Apple-Cinnamon Cauliflower Porridge

Prep Time: 10 minutes | **Cook Time:** 15 minutes | **Servings:** 4

Ingredients:

- 1 medium head of cauliflower, riced
- 1 medium apple, peeled and diced
- 1 cup full-fat coconut milk
- 1/2 cup water
- 1 tablespoon coconut oil
- 1 teaspoon ground cinnamon
- 1/4 teaspoon ground ginger
- 1/4 teaspoon ground cloves
- 1/4 teaspoon sea salt

Instructions:

1. In a large saucepan, heat the coconut oil over medium heat. Add the peeled and diced apple and cook until softened, about 5 minutes.

2. Add the riced cauliflower to the saucepan with the apple. Stir to combine.

3. Pour in the full-fat coconut milk and water, stirring to mix adequately.

4. Add the ground cinnamon, ground ginger, ground cloves, and sea salt to the mixture. Stir to combine.

5. Bring the mixture to a gentle simmer. Cook, stirring occasionally, until the cauliflower is tender and the porridge has thickened, about 10 minutes.

6. Remove from heat and let it cool slightly before serving.

Nutritional Information (per serving):

- **Calories:** 170 kcal
- **Fat:** 12 g
- **Carbohydrates:** 14 g
- **Proteins:** 3 g

Breakfast Sausage Patties with Sautéed Greens

Prep Time: 15 minutes | **Cook Time:** 20 minutes | **Servings:** 4

Ingredients:

- **For the Sausage Patties:**

  - 1-pound ground pork (AIP-compliant, no additives)
  - 1 teaspoon dried thyme
  - 1 teaspoon dried sage
  - 1/2 teaspoon ground ginger
  - 1/2 teaspoon sea salt
  - 1/4 teaspoon ground cloves
  - 1/4 teaspoon ground cinnamon

- **For the Sautéed Greens:**

  - 1 bunch kale, stems removed and chopped
  - 2 cloves garlic, minced
  - 2 tablespoons coconut oil
  - 1/2 teaspoon sea salt
  - 1/4 teaspoon ground black pepper (optional, AIP reintroduction phase)
  - 1 tablespoon apple cider vinegar

Instructions:

1. In a large bowl, combine the ground pork, dried thyme, dried sage, ground ginger, sea salt, ground cloves, and ground cinnamon. Mix adequately to incorporate the spices evenly.

2. Form the mixture into 8 small patties.

3. Heat a large skillet over medium heat and add the sausage patties. Cook for about 4-5 minutes on each side, or until fully cooked through. Take out the patties from the skillet and set aside.

4. In the same skillet, heat the coconut oil over medium heat.

5. Add the minced garlic and cook for about 1 minute until fragrant.

6. Add the chopped kale, sea salt, and optional ground black pepper. Cook, stirring frequently, until the kale is wilted and tender, about 5-7 minutes.

7. Stir in the apple cider vinegar and cook for an additional 1-2 minutes.

8. Serve the sausage patties hot with the sautéed greens on the side.

Nutritional Information (per serving):

- **Calories:** 280 kcal
- **Fat:** 20 g
- **Carbohydrates:** 6 g
- **Proteins:** 18 g

Coconut Yogurt with Blueberries and Honey

Prep Time: 5 minutes | **Cook Time:** 0 minutes | **Servings:** 4

Ingredients:

- 2 cups coconut yogurt (AIP-compliant)
- 1 cup fresh blueberries
- 2 tablespoons honey
- 1 teaspoon ground cinnamon (optional)

Instructions:

1. Divide the coconut yogurt evenly among four serving bowls.
2. Top each serving with 1/4 cup of fresh blueberries.
3. Drizzle each bowl with 1/2 tablespoon of honey.
4. Sprinkle with ground cinnamon if desired.

Nutritional Information (per serving):

- **Calories:** 180 kcal
- **Fat:** 9 g
  - **Monounsaturated Fat:** 1 g
  - **Polyunsaturated Fat:** 0.5 g
- **Carbohydrates:** 22 g
- **Proteins:** 2 g

AIP Pumpkin Pancakes with Maple Syrup

Prep Time: 10 minutes | **Cook Time:** 20 minutes | **Servings:** 4

Ingredients:

- 1 cup pumpkin puree
- 1/2 cup coconut milk
- 1/4 cup coconut flour
- 1/4 cup arrowroot flour
- 1 tablespoon maple syrup (plus extra for serving)
- 1 teaspoon ground cinnamon
- 1/2 teaspoon ground ginger
- 1/4 teaspoon ground cloves
- 1/4 teaspoon sea salt
- 1/4 teaspoon baking soda
- 2 tablespoons coconut oil (for cooking)

Instructions:

1. In a large mixing bowl, combine the pumpkin puree, coconut milk, and 1 tablespoon of maple syrup. Mix until well combined.
2. Add the coconut flour, arrowroot flour, ground cinnamon, ground ginger, ground cloves, sea salt, and baking soda to the wet ingredients. Stir until a batter forms.
3. Heat 1/2 tablespoon of coconut oil in a large skillet over medium heat.
4. Scoop 1/4 cup of batter into the skillet for each pancake, spreading it slightly with the back of a spoon. Cook for 3-4 minutes until the edges are set and bubbles form on the surface.
5. Carefully flip the pancake and cook for an additional 2-3 minutes until golden brown and cooked through.
6. Repeat with the remaining batter, adding more coconut oil to the skillet as needed.
7. Serve the pancakes hot, drizzled with additional maple syrup.

Nutritional Information (per serving):

- **Calories:** 210 kcal
- **Fat:** 14 g
  - **Monounsaturated Fat:** 2 g
  - **Polyunsaturated Fat:** 1 g
- **Carbohydrates:** 19 g
- **Proteins:** 3 g

Banana and Coconut Smoothie

Prep Time: 5 minutes | **Cook Time:** 0 minutes | **Servings:** 2

Ingredients:

- 2 ripe bananas, sliced

- 1 cup coconut milk

- 1/2 cup water

- 1 tablespoon coconut oil

- 1 teaspoon ground cinnamon

- 1/2 teaspoon vanilla extract (AIP-compliant)

Instructions:

1. Place the sliced bananas, coconut milk, water, coconut oil, ground cinnamon, and vanilla extract in a blender.

2. Blend on high until smooth and creamy.

3. Pour the smoothie into two glasses and serve immediately.

Nutritional Information (per serving):

- **Calories:** 210 kcal

- **Fat:** 14 g

  - **Monounsaturated Fat:** 1 g

  - **Polyunsaturated Fat:** 0.5 g

- **Carbohydrates:** 23 g

- **Proteins:** 2 g

Carrot and Parsnip Hash Browns

Prep Time: 10 minutes | **Cook Time:** 20 minutes | **Servings:** 4

Ingredients:

- 2 large carrots, peeled and grated
- 2 large parsnips, peeled and grated
- 1/4 cup green onions, finely chopped
- 1/4 cup arrowroot flour
- 1/2 teaspoon sea salt
- 1/4 teaspoon ground black pepper (optional, AIP reintroduction phase)
- 2 tablespoons coconut oil

Instructions:

1. In a large bowl, combine the peeled and grated carrots, peeled and grated parsnips, and finely chopped green onions.
2. Add the arrowroot flour, sea salt, and optional ground black pepper. Mix adequately to combine.
3. Heat 1 tablespoon of coconut oil in a large skillet over medium heat.
4. Scoop about 1/4 cup of the vegetable mixture into the skillet, flattening it slightly to form a patty. Repeat with the remaining mixture, cooking the hash browns in batches.
5. Cook each hash brown for about 3-4 minutes per side, until golden brown and crispy.
6. Take out the hash browns from the skillet and place them on a paper towel-lined plate to drain any excess oil.
7. Add the remaining 1 tablespoon of coconut oil to the skillet as needed for cooking the rest of the hash browns.
8. Serve the hash browns hot.

Nutritional Information (per serving):

- **Calories:** 150 kcal
- **Fat:** 9 g
- **Carbohydrates:** 17 g
- **Proteins:** 1 g

Smoked Salmon and Avocado Salad

Prep Time: 15 minutes | **Cook Time:** 0 minutes | **Servings:** 2

Ingredients:

- 6 ounces smoked salmon, thinly sliced
- 1 avocado, sliced
- 2 cups mixed greens (AIP-compliant)
- 1/4 cup cucumber, thinly sliced
- 1/4 cup red onion, thinly sliced
- 1 tablespoon fresh dill, chopped
- 1 tablespoon extra virgin olive oil
- 1 tablespoon lemon juice
- Sea salt, to taste
- Ground black pepper (optional, AIP reintroduction phase)

Instructions:

1. In a large bowl, combine the mixed greens, thinly sliced cucumber, thinly sliced red onion, and chopped fresh dill.

2. Drizzle the extra virgin olive oil and lemon juice over the salad ingredients. Season with sea salt and optional ground black pepper to taste. Toss gently to combine.

3. Divide the salad mixture evenly between two plates.

4. Top each plate with sliced avocado and smoked salmon.

5. Serve immediately.

Nutritional Information (per serving):

- **Calories:** 320 kcal
- **Fat:** 22 g
  - **Monounsaturated Fat:** 10 g
  - **Polyunsaturated Fat:** 3 g
- **Carbohydrates:** 15 g
- **Proteins:** 18 g

Cauliflower Rice Breakfast Bowl

Prep Time: 10 minutes | **Cook Time:** 10 minutes | **Servings:** 2

Ingredients:

- 1 small head cauliflower, grated into rice-like pieces
- 1 tablespoon coconut oil
- 4 slices bacon, chopped (AIP-compliant)
- 2 cups baby spinach
- 1 avocado, sliced
- 4 large eggs
- Sea salt, to taste
- Ground black pepper (optional, AIP reintroduction phase)
- Fresh herbs, for garnish (optional)

Instructions:

1. Heat the coconut oil in a large skillet over medium heat.
2. Add the chopped bacon and cook until crispy.
3. Add the grated cauliflower rice to the skillet. Cook, stirring frequently, until the cauliflower is tender, about 5-7 minutes.
4. Meanwhile, in a separate pan, fry the eggs to your desired doneness.
5. Once the cauliflower rice is cooked, stir in the baby spinach until wilted.
6. Divide the cauliflower rice and spinach mixture between two bowls.
7. Top each bowl with sliced avocado and fried eggs.
8. Season with sea salt and optional ground black pepper.
9. Garnish with fresh herbs if desired.
10. Serve hot.

Nutritional Information (per serving):

- **Calories:** 420 kcal
- **Fat:** 30 g
  - **Monounsaturated Fat:** 12 g
  - **Polyunsaturated Fat:** 4 g
- **Carbohydrates:** 16 g
- **Proteins:** 22 g

Chicken Apple Breakfast Meatballs

Prep Time: 15 minutes | **Cook Time:** 20 minutes | **Servings:** 4

Ingredients:

- 1-pound ground chicken
- 1 medium apple, peeled and grated
- 1/4 cup finely chopped onion
- 2 tablespoons fresh parsley, finely chopped
- 1 teaspoon dried sage
- 1/2 teaspoon sea salt
- 1/4 teaspoon ground black pepper (optional, AIP reintroduction phase)
- 1 tablespoon coconut oil

Instructions:

1. Preheat the oven to 400°F (200°C). Line a baking sheet with parchment paper.
2. In a large bowl, combine the ground chicken, grated apple, finely chopped onion, chopped parsley, dried sage, sea salt, and optional ground black pepper.
3. Mix the ingredients until well combined.
4. Scoop about 1 tablespoon of the mixture and roll it into a ball. Repeat with the remaining mixture, forming meatballs.
5. Heat the coconut oil in a large skillet over medium-high heat.
6. Brown the meatballs on all sides, working in batches if necessary, for about 2-3 minutes per side.
7. Transfer the browned meatballs to the prepared baking sheet.
8. Bake in the preheated oven for 12-15 minutes, or until cooked through and no longer pink in the center.
9. Remove from the oven and let cool slightly before serving.

Nutritional Information (per serving):

- **Calories:** 280 kcal
- **Fat:** 16 g
    - **Monounsaturated Fat:** 6 g
    - **Polyunsaturated Fat:** 2 g
- **Carbohydrates:** 7 g
- **Proteins:** 26 g

Butternut Squash and Sage Breakfast Skillet

Prep Time: 15 minutes | **Cook Time:** 25 minutes | **Servings:** 4

Ingredients:

- 1 small butternut squash, peeled, seeded, and diced
- 1 tablespoon coconut oil
- 1 onion, diced
- 2 cloves garlic, minced
- 1 tablespoon fresh sage leaves, chopped
- 8 ounces ground turkey
- Sea salt, to taste
- Ground black pepper (optional, AIP reintroduction phase)
- Fresh parsley, chopped, for garnish (optional)

Instructions:

1. Heat the coconut oil in a large skillet over medium heat.
2. Add the diced butternut squash and cook, stirring occasionally, until slightly tender, about 8-10 minutes.
3. Add the diced onion to the skillet and cook until translucent, about 5 minutes.
4. Stir in the minced garlic and chopped sage leaves, cooking for another 1-2 minutes until fragrant.
5. Push the vegetables to the side of the skillet and add the ground turkey. Cook, breaking it apart with a spatula, until browned and cooked through, about 5-7 minutes.
6. Season with sea salt and optional ground black pepper to taste.
7. Remove from heat and garnish with chopped fresh parsley if desired.
8. Serve hot.

Nutritional Information (per serving):

- **Calories:** 250 kcal
- **Fat:** 10 g
  - **Monounsaturated Fat:** 4 g
  - **Polyunsaturated Fat:** 2 g
- **Carbohydrates:** 30 g
- **Proteins:** 15 g

Lunch Recipes

Zucchini Noodles with Ground Turkey and Avocado Pesto

Prep Time: 15 minutes | **Cook Time:** 20 minutes | **Number of Servings:** 4

Ingredients:

For the Zucchini Noodles:

- 4 medium zucchinis, spiralized

For the Ground Turkey:

- 1-pound ground turkey, lean

For the Avocado Pesto:

- 2 ripe avocados, peeled and pitted
- 1/4 cup fresh basil leaves, chopped
- 2 tablespoons extra virgin olive oil
- 1 tablespoon lemon juice
- 1 garlic clove, minced
- Sea salt, to taste
- Freshly ground black pepper, to taste

Optional Garnishes:

- Fresh basil leaves, chopped
- Zest of 1 lemon

Instructions:

1. Using a spiralizer, create noodles from the zucchinis. Set aside.

2. In a large skillet over medium heat, add the ground turkey. Break it apart with a spatula. Cook until browned and cooked through, about 5-7 minutes. Season with sea salt and freshly ground black pepper to taste. Remove from heat and set aside.

3. In a blender or food processor, combine the avocados, chopped basil leaves, extra virgin olive oil, lemon juice, minced garlic, sea salt, and black pepper. Blend until smooth and creamy.

4. Add the zucchini noodles to the skillet with the cooked ground turkey. Toss to combine and heat through, about 2 minutes. Pour the avocado pesto over the zucchini noodles and turkey, tossing until evenly coated. Serve warm, garnished with fresh basil leaves and lemon zest, if desired.

Nutritional Information (per serving):

- **Calories:** 350 kcal
- **Fat:** 22 g
- **Carbohydrates:** 14 g
- **Proteins:** 28 g

Chicken and Vegetable Soup

Prep Time: 15 minutes | **Cook Time:** 30 minutes | **Number of Servings:** 6

Ingredients:

For the Soup:

- 1 tablespoon coconut oil
- 1 onion, diced
- 3 cloves garlic, minced
- 3 carrots, peeled and diced
- 3 celery stalks, diced
- 1 medium turnip, peeled and diced
- 1-pound boneless, skinless chicken breasts, diced

- 6 cups bone broth or chicken broth
- 1 teaspoon dried thyme
- 1 teaspoon dried parsley
- Sea salt, to taste
- Freshly ground black pepper, to taste
- Fresh parsley, chopped (for garnish)

Instructions:

1. In a large pot, heat coconut oil over medium heat. Add diced onion and minced garlic. Sauté until onion becomes translucent, about 3-4 minutes.

2. Add diced carrots, celery, and turnip to the pot. Sauté for another 5 minutes, stirring occasionally. Add diced chicken breasts and cook until chicken is no longer pink, about 5 minutes more.

3. Pour in bone broth or chicken broth into the pot. Add dried thyme and dried parsley. Season with sea salt and freshly ground black pepper to taste. Bring the soup to a boil, then reduce heat to low. Cover and simmer for 15-20 minutes, or until vegetables are tender and chicken is cooked through.

4. Ladle the soup into bowls. Garnish with freshly chopped parsley. Serve hot.

Nutritional Information (per serving):

- **Calories:** 240 kcal
- **Fat:** 8 g
- **Carbohydrates:** 12 g
- **Proteins:** 28 g

Tuna Salad Lettuce Wraps

Prep Time: 15 minutes | **Cook Time:** 0 minutes | **Number of Servings:** 4

Ingredients:

For the Tuna Salad:

- 2 cans (5 ounces each) tuna, drained
- 1/2 cup finely diced cucumber
- 1/4 cup finely diced red onion
- 1/4 cup finely chopped fresh parsley
- 2 tablespoons olive oil
- 2 tablespoons lemon juice
- Sea salt, to taste
- Freshly ground black pepper, to taste

For Wrapping:

- 8 large lettuce leaves (such as butter lettuce or romaine)

Instructions:

1. In a mixing bowl, combine drained tuna, finely diced cucumber, finely diced red onion, chopped fresh parsley, olive oil, and lemon juice. Mix adequately to combine. Season with sea salt and freshly ground black pepper to taste.

2. Lay out the lettuce leaves on a clean surface. Spoon the tuna salad mixture evenly onto each lettuce leaf.

3. Roll up each lettuce leaf around the tuna salad mixture, securing the wraps with toothpicks if needed. Serve immediately.

Nutritional Information (per serving):

- **Calories:** 180 kcal
- **Fat:** 9 g
- **Carbohydrates:** 4 g
- **Proteins:** 20 g

Shrimp and Mango Salad

Prep Time: 15 minutes | **Cook Time:** 5 minutes | **Number of Servings:** 4

Ingredients:

For the Salad:

- 1-pound shrimp, peeled and deveined
- 2 ripe mangoes, peeled, pitted, and diced
- 1 cucumber, peeled, seeded, and diced
- 1/4 cup red onion, finely chopped
- 1/4 cup fresh cilantro leaves, chopped

For the Dressing:

- 2 tablespoons olive oil
- 2 tablespoons lime juice
- 1 tablespoon honey (substitute with AIP-compliant sweetener if necessary)
- Sea salt, to taste
- Freshly ground black pepper, to taste

Instructions:

1. In a large skillet over medium heat, cook the shrimp for about 2-3 minutes per side, or until pink and opaque. Remove from heat and let cool slightly.

2. In a large bowl, combine the diced mangoes, diced cucumber, finely chopped red onion, and chopped cilantro.

3. In a small bowl, whisk together the olive oil, lime juice, honey (or AIP-compliant sweetener), sea salt, and freshly ground black pepper.

4. Add the cooked shrimp to the bowl with the mango mixture. Pour the dressing over the salad and gently toss to combine, ensuring everything is evenly coated.

5. Divide the salad into individual servings. Optionally, garnish with additional cilantro leaves. Serve immediately.

Nutritional Information (per serving):

- **Calories:** 280 kcal
- **Fat:** 10 g
- **Carbohydrates:** 24 g
- **Proteins:** 25 g

Beef and Broccoli Stir-fry

Prep Time: 15 minutes | **Cook Time:** 15 minutes | **Number of Servings:** 4

Ingredients:

For the Stir-fry:

- 1-pound flank steak, thinly sliced across the grain
- 1 head broccoli, cut into florets
- 1 carrot, thinly sliced
- 1 bell pepper, thinly sliced
- 3 cloves garlic, minced
- 1-inch piece of ginger, peeled and minced

- 2 tablespoons coconut aminos (AIP substitute for soy sauce)
- 1 tablespoon olive oil
- Sea salt, to taste
- Freshly ground black pepper, to taste
- Fresh cilantro leaves, chopped (for garnish)

Instructions:

1. Season the thinly sliced flank steak with sea salt and freshly ground black pepper.

2. Heat olive oil in a large skillet or wok over medium-high heat. Add minced garlic and minced ginger, stirring for about 30 seconds until fragrant. Add thinly sliced carrots and bell pepper, stir-frying for about 2-3 minutes until slightly tender.

3. Push the vegetables to the side of the skillet. Add the seasoned flank steak slices in a single layer. Cook for about 2-3 minutes on each side until browned and cooked to desired doneness.

4. Add broccoli florets to the skillet. Pour in coconut aminos and stir-fry for another 2-3 minutes, or until the broccoli is tender-crisp and the beef is fully cooked.

5. Garnish with chopped fresh cilantro leaves. Serve hot, optionally over cauliflower rice for a complete meal.

Nutritional Information (per serving):

- **Calories:** 320 kcal
- **Fat:** 15 g
- **Carbohydrates:** 10 g
- **Proteins:** 35 g

AIP Caesar Salad with Grilled Chicken

Prep Time: 20 minutes | **Cook Time:** 15 minutes | **Number of Servings:** 4

Ingredients:

For the Salad:

- 1-pound chicken breasts, boneless and skinless
- 1 head romaine lettuce, chopped
- 1/2 cucumber, sliced
- 1 avocado, sliced
- 1/4 cup chopped fresh parsley (for garnish)

For the Dressing:

- 1/2 cup coconut milk (full-fat, canned)
- 2 tablespoons olive oil
- 2 tablespoons lemon juice
- 1 tablespoon apple cider vinegar
- 1 tablespoon nutritional yeast (optional, for cheesy flavor)
- 1 clove garlic, minced
- Sea salt, to taste
- Freshly ground black pepper, to taste (omit for strict AIP)

Instructions:

1. Preheat a grill or grill pan over medium-high heat. Season the chicken breasts with sea salt and freshly ground black pepper (if using). Grill for about 6-7 minutes per side, or until fully cooked through and grill marks appear. Remove from heat and let rest for 5 minutes before slicing.

2. In a blender or food processor, combine coconut milk, olive oil, lemon juice, apple cider vinegar, nutritional yeast (if using), minced garlic, sea salt, and freshly ground black pepper (if using). Blend until smooth and creamy. Adjust seasoning to taste.

3. In a large bowl, toss the chopped romaine lettuce with sliced cucumber and avocado slices.

4. Divide the salad onto plates. Top each serving with grilled chicken slices. Drizzle the creamy Caesar dressing over the salads. Garnish with chopped fresh parsley.

5. Serve immediately and enjoy your AIP-friendly Caesar salad with grilled chicken!

Nutritional Information (per serving):

- **Calories:** 320 kcal
- **Fat:** 20 g
- **Carbohydrates:** 10 g
- **Proteins:** 25 g

Turkey and Apple Slaw

Prep Time: 15 minutes | **Cook Time:** 0 minutes | **Number of Servings:** 4

Ingredients:

For the Slaw:

- 1-pound turkey breast, cooked and shredded
- 2 cups shredded green cabbage
- 1 cup shredded red cabbage
- 1 large apple, thinly sliced
- 1/4 cup chopped fresh parsley
- 1/4 cup chopped green onions

For the Dressing:

- 1/4 cup olive oil
- 2 tablespoons apple cider vinegar
- 1 tablespoon honey (substitute with AIP-compliant sweetener if necessary)
- 1 teaspoon Dijon mustard (check for AIP compliance or omit)
- Sea salt, to taste
- Freshly ground black pepper, to taste (omit for strict AIP)

Instructions:

1. In a large bowl, combine shredded green cabbage, shredded red cabbage, thinly sliced apple, chopped fresh parsley, and chopped green onions.

2. In a small bowl, whisk together olive oil, apple cider vinegar, honey (or AIP-compliant sweetener), Dijon mustard (if using), sea salt, and freshly ground black pepper (if using).

3. Add the cooked and shredded turkey breast to the bowl with the slaw ingredients.

4. Pour the dressing over the turkey and slaw mixture. Toss gently until everything is well coated with the dressing.

5. Divide the turkey and apple slaw onto plates or bowls. Serve immediately.

Nutritional Information (per serving):

- **Calories:** 280 kcal
- **Fat:** 15 g
- **Carbohydrates:** 12 g
- **Proteins:** 25 g

Salmon Salad with Cucumber and Dill

Prep Time: 15 minutes | **Cook Time:** 15 minutes | **Number of Servings:** 4

Ingredients:

For the Salmon:

- 1-pound salmon fillets, skinless
- 1 tablespoon olive oil
- Sea salt, to taste
- Freshly ground black pepper, to taste

For the Salad:

- 1 English cucumber, thinly sliced
- 1/4 cup fresh dill, chopped
- 1/4 cup red onion, thinly sliced
- 1 avocado, diced

For the Dressing:

- 1/4 cup olive oil
- 2 tablespoons lemon juice
- 1 tablespoon Dijon mustard (check for AIP compliance or omit)
- Sea salt, to taste
- Freshly ground black pepper, to taste (omit for strict AIP)

Instructions:

1. Preheat the oven to 400°F (200°C). Place the salmon fillets on a baking sheet lined with parchment paper. Drizzle olive oil over the salmon and season with sea salt and freshly ground black pepper. Bake for 12-15 minutes, or until the salmon is cooked through and flakes easily with a fork. Remove from the oven and let cool slightly.

2. In a small bowl, whisk together olive oil, lemon juice, Dijon mustard (if using), sea salt, and freshly ground black pepper (if using).

3. In a large bowl, combine thinly sliced cucumber, chopped fresh dill, thinly sliced red onion, and diced avocado.

4. Flake the baked salmon into bite-sized pieces and add to the bowl with the salad ingredients.

5. Pour the dressing over the salad and salmon mixture. Gently toss until everything is well coated with the dressing.

6. Divide the salmon salad onto plates or bowls. Serve immediately.

Nutritional Information (per serving):

- **Calories:** 320 kcal
- **Fat:** 20 g
- **Carbohydrates:** 10 g
- **Proteins:** 25 g

AIP Cobb Salad with Balsamic Dressing

Prep Time: 20 minutes | **Cook Time:** 15 minutes | **Number of Servings:** 4

Ingredients:

For the Salad:

- 1-pound chicken breasts, boneless and skinless
- 6 cups mixed greens (such as romaine lettuce and spinach)
- 1 avocado, diced
- 1 cucumber, diced
- 2 medium beets, roasted and diced (AIP substitute for traditional Cobb salad ingredients)
- 4 slices cooked bacon, crumbled (check for AIP compliance or omit)
- 1/4 cup chopped fresh chives

For the Balsamic Dressing:

- 1/4 cup olive oil
- 2 tablespoons balsamic vinegar
- 1 teaspoon honey (substitute with AIP-compliant sweetener if necessary)
- Sea salt, to taste
- Freshly ground black pepper, to taste (omit for strict AIP)

Instructions:

1. Preheat the oven to 400°F (200°C). Place the chicken breasts on a baking sheet lined with parchment paper. Drizzle with olive oil and season with sea salt and freshly ground black pepper. Bake for 15-20 minutes, or until the chicken is cooked through and no longer pink in the center. Remove from the oven and let cool slightly before slicing.

2. In a small bowl, whisk together olive oil, balsamic vinegar, honey (or AIP-compliant sweetener), sea salt, and freshly ground black pepper (if using).

3. Arrange the mixed greens in a large salad bowl or divide among individual plates. Top with diced avocado, diced cucumber, roasted and diced beets, crumbled bacon (if using), and chopped fresh chives.

4. Slice the baked chicken breasts and arrange on top of the salad.

5. Drizzle the balsamic dressing over the salad.

6. Serve the AIP Cobb salad immediately.

Nutritional Information (per serving):

- **Calories:** 320 kcal
- **Fat:** 18 g
- **Carbohydrates:** 15 g
- **Proteins:** 25 g

<u>Grilled Chicken with Mixed Greens and Lemon Vinaigrette</u>

Prep Time: 15 minutes | **Cook Time:** 15 minutes | **Number of Servings:** 4

Ingredients:

For the Grilled Chicken:

- 1-pound chicken breasts, boneless and skinless
- 1 tablespoon olive oil
- Sea salt, to taste
- Freshly ground black pepper, to taste

For the Salad:

- 6 cups mixed greens (such as spinach, arugula, and kale)
- 1 cucumber, thinly sliced
- 1 cup cherry tomatoes, halved
- 1/4 cup thinly sliced red onion

For the Lemon Vinaigrette:

- 1/4 cup olive oil
- 2 tablespoons fresh lemon juice
- 1 teaspoon Dijon mustard (check for AIP compliance or omit)
- 1 clove garlic, minced
- Sea salt, to taste
- Freshly ground black pepper, to taste (omit for strict AIP)

Instructions:

1. Preheat a grill or grill pan over medium-high heat. Brush the chicken breasts with olive oil and season with sea salt and freshly ground black pepper. Grill for about 6-7 minutes per side, or until the chicken is cooked through and no longer pink in the center. Remove from heat and let rest for 5 minutes before slicing.

2. In a small bowl, whisk together olive oil, fresh lemon juice, Dijon mustard (if using), minced garlic, sea salt, and freshly ground black pepper (if using).

3. In a large salad bowl, combine mixed greens, thinly sliced cucumber, cherry tomatoes, and thinly sliced red onion.

4. Slice the grilled chicken breasts into thin strips.

5. Add the sliced grilled chicken to the salad bowl. Drizzle the lemon vinaigrette over the salad and chicken. Toss gently to combine and coat everything with the dressing.

6. Divide the grilled chicken salad onto plates. Serve immediately.

Nutritional Information (per serving):

- **Calories:** 280 kcal
- **Fat:** 18 g
- **Carbohydrates:** 10 g
- **Proteins:** 25 g

AIP BLT Salad with Avocado Dressing

Prep Time: 20 minutes | **Cook Time:** 10 minutes | **Number of Servings:** 4

Ingredients:

For the Salad:

- 1-pound nitrate-free bacon (check for AIP compliance)
- 6 cups mixed greens (such as spinach and romaine lettuce)
- 1 cucumber, diced
- 1 avocado, diced
- 1/4 cup chopped fresh chives

For the Avocado Dressing:

- 1 ripe avocado, peeled and pitted
- 1/4 cup coconut milk (full-fat, canned)
- 2 tablespoons fresh lemon juice
- 1 tablespoon extra virgin olive oil
- Sea salt, to taste
- Freshly ground black pepper, to taste (omit for strict AIP)

Instructions:

1. In a skillet over medium heat, cook the bacon until crispy. Transfer to a paper towel-lined plate to drain excess fat. Once cooled, crumble or chop the bacon into small pieces.

2. In a blender or food processor, combine the ripe avocado, coconut milk, fresh lemon juice, extra virgin olive oil, sea salt, and freshly ground black pepper (if using). Blend until smooth and creamy. Adjust seasoning to taste.

3. In a large salad bowl, combine the mixed greens, diced cucumber, diced avocado, chopped fresh chives, and crumbled bacon.

4. Pour the avocado dressing over the salad ingredients.

5. Gently toss the salad to coat everything evenly with the avocado dressing.

6. Divide the AIP BLT salad onto plates and serve immediately.

Nutritional Information (per serving):

- **Calories:** 380 kcal
- **Fat:** 28 g
- **Carbohydrates:** 15 g
- **Proteins:** 18 g

Roasted Vegetable and Herb Salad

Prep Time: 15 minutes | **Cook Time:** 30 minutes | **Number of Servings:** 4

Ingredients:

For the Salad:

- 1 large sweet potato, peeled and diced
- 2 carrots, peeled and sliced into rounds
- 1 large zucchini, diced
- 1 red bell pepper, seeded and diced
- 1 yellow bell pepper, seeded and diced
- 1/2 red onion, thinly sliced
- 2 tablespoons olive oil
- Sea salt, to taste
- Freshly ground black pepper, to taste
- 4 cups mixed greens (such as spinach and arugula)
- 1/4 cup chopped fresh parsley
- 1/4 cup chopped fresh basil
- 1/4 cup chopped fresh cilantro

For the Dressing:

- 3 tablespoons extra virgin olive oil
- 2 tablespoons fresh lemon juice
- 1 teaspoon honey (optional, omit for strict AIP)
- Sea salt, to taste
- Freshly ground black pepper, to taste (omit for strict AIP)

Instructions:

1. Preheat the oven to 400°F (200°C). Line a baking sheet with parchment paper.

2. In a large bowl, toss the diced sweet potato, sliced carrots, diced zucchini, diced red bell pepper, diced yellow bell pepper, and thinly sliced red onion with olive oil, sea salt, and freshly ground black pepper.

3. Spread the vegetables evenly on the prepared baking sheet. Roast in the preheated oven for 25-30 minutes, or until the vegetables are tender and lightly browned, stirring halfway through cooking.

4. In a small bowl, whisk together extra virgin olive oil, fresh lemon juice, honey (if using), sea salt, and freshly ground black pepper (if using).

5. In a large salad bowl, combine the roasted vegetables with mixed greens, chopped fresh parsley, chopped fresh basil, and chopped fresh cilantro. Next, pour the dressing over the salad ingredients.

6. Gently toss the salad to coat everything evenly with the dressing.

7. Divide the roasted vegetable and herb salad onto plates and serve immediately.

Nutritional Information (per serving):

- **Calories:** 280 kcal
- **Fat:** 18 g
- **Carbohydrates:** 28 g
- **Proteins:** 5 g

Dinner Recipes

Baked Salmon with Asparagus and Mashed Cauliflower

Prep Time: 15 minutes | **Cook Time:** 25 minutes | **Servings:** 4

Ingredients:

- 4 salmon fillets
- 1 bunch asparagus, trimmed
- 1 head cauliflower, chopped into florets
- 3 cloves garlic, minced
-

- 2 tablespoons olive oil
- Salt and pepper, to taste
- Fresh dill, for garnish (optional)

Instructions:

1. Preheat the oven to 400°F (200°C). Line a baking sheet with parchment paper.
2. Steam the cauliflower florets until very tender, about 10-12 minutes.
3. Drain the cauliflower and transfer to a large bowl. Mash with a potato masher or blend until smooth. Season with salt and pepper to taste.
4. Toss the trimmed asparagus with 1 tablespoon of olive oil, minced garlic, salt, and pepper on the prepared baking sheet.
5. Arrange the salmon fillets on the baking sheet with the asparagus. Drizzle the remaining olive oil over the salmon. Season with salt and pepper.
6. Bake in the preheated oven for 12-15 minutes, or until salmon is cooked through and flakes easily with a fork.
7. Serve the baked salmon and asparagus alongside the mashed cauliflower.
8. Garnish with fresh dill if desired.

Nutritional Information (per serving):

- **Calories:** 320 kcal
- **Fat:** 17g
- **Carbohydrates:** 10g
- **Protein:** 31g

Braised Lamb Shanks with Root Vegetables

Prep Time: 20 minutes | **Cook Time:** 2 hours 30 minutes | **Servings:** 4

Ingredients:

- 4 lamb shanks
- 2 carrots, peeled and sliced
- 2 parsnips, peeled and sliced
- 1 celery root (celeriac), peeled and diced
- 1 onion, diced
- 4 cloves garlic, minced
- 2 cups bone broth or beef broth (check for AIP compliance)
- 1 tablespoon apple cider vinegar
- 2 tablespoons olive oil
- Salt and pepper, to taste
- Fresh parsley, for garnish (optional)

Instructions:

1. Preheat the oven to 325°F (160°C).
2. Season the lamb shanks generously with salt and pepper.
3. In a large Dutch oven or oven-safe pot, heat 1 tablespoon of olive oil over medium-high heat. Brown the lamb shanks on all sides, about 8-10 minutes total. Remove and set aside.
4. In the same pot, add the remaining olive oil if needed. Add the diced onion, minced garlic, carrots, parsnips, and celery root. Sauté for 5-7 minutes until slightly softened.
5. Pour in the bone broth and apple cider vinegar, scraping up any browned bits from the bottom of the pot.
6. Return the lamb shanks to the pot, nestling them among the vegetables. Bring to a simmer.
7. Cover the pot with a lid and transfer to the preheated oven. Braise for 2 to 2 1/2 hours, or until the lamb is tender and easily pulls away from the bone.
8. Remove from the oven. Serve the lamb shanks with the braised root vegetables.
9. Garnish with fresh parsley if desired.

Nutritional Information (per serving):

- **Calories:** 480 kcal
- **Fat:** 27g
- **Carbohydrates:** 12g
- **Protein:** 45g

AIP Meatloaf with Sweet Potato Mash

Prep Time: 20 minutes | **Cook Time:** 1 hour | **Servings:** 4

Ingredients:

For the Meatloaf:

- 1-pound ground beef (preferably grass-fed)
- 1-pound ground pork
- 1 onion, finely diced
- 2 cloves garlic, minced
- 1/2 cup chopped fresh parsley
- 1/4 cup coconut flour
- 1/4 cup coconut milk (full-fat, canned)
- 1 tablespoon apple cider vinegar
- 1 teaspoon dried thyme
- 1 teaspoon dried oregano
- Salt and pepper, to taste

For the Sweet Potato Mash:

- 2 large sweet potatoes, peeled and cubed
- 2 tablespoons coconut oil
- Salt, to taste
- Fresh chives, chopped (for garnish, optional)

Instructions:

1. Preheat the oven to 375°F (190°C). Grease a loaf pan with coconut oil or line it with parchment paper.
2. In a large mixing bowl, combine ground beef, ground pork, diced onion, minced garlic, chopped parsley, coconut flour, coconut milk, apple cider vinegar, dried thyme, dried oregano, salt, and pepper. Mix until well combined.
3. Transfer the mixture to the prepared loaf pan, pressing it evenly into the pan.
4. Bake in the preheated oven for 45-50 minutes, or until the internal temperature reaches 160°F (71°C) and the top is nicely browned.
5. While the meatloaf is baking, place the sweet potato cubes in a large pot and cover with water. Bring to a boil over medium-high heat.
6. Reduce heat to medium-low and simmer for 15-20 minutes, or until the sweet potatoes are fork-tender.
7. Drain the sweet potatoes and return them to the pot. Add coconut oil and season with salt. Mash until smooth.
8. Slice the meatloaf and serve with a generous portion of sweet potato mash.
9. Garnish with chopped fresh chives if desired.

Nutritional Information (per serving):

- **Calories:** 580 kcal
- **Fat:** 34g
- **Carbohydrates:** 30g
- **Protein:** 39g

Coconut-Crusted Cod with Steamed Broccoli

Prep Time: 15 minutes | **Cook Time:** 15 minutes | **Servings:** 4

Ingredients:

For the Coconut-Crusted Cod:

- 4 cod fillets (about 6 ounces each)
- 1/2 cup coconut flour
- 1/2 cup shredded coconut (unsweetened)
- 2 eggs, beaten
- 1/4 cup coconut milk (full-fat, canned)
- 1/2 teaspoon garlic powder
- Salt and pepper, to taste
- Coconut oil, for frying

For the Steamed Broccoli:

- 1 head broccoli, cut into florets
- Lemon wedges, for serving (optional)

Instructions:

1. Pat the cod fillets dry with paper towels.
2. In one shallow bowl, place coconut flour. In another shallow bowl, combine shredded coconut, garlic powder, salt, and pepper.
3. In a third bowl, whisk together beaten eggs and coconut milk.
4. Dredge each cod fillet in coconut flour, shaking off excess. Dip into the egg mixture, allowing excess to drip off. Press into the shredded coconut mixture, ensuring the fillet is evenly coated.
5. Heat coconut oil in a large skillet over medium-high heat. Fry the cod fillets for about 3-4 minutes per side, until golden brown and cooked through. Transfer to a plate lined with paper towels to drain excess oil.
6. While the cod is cooking, steam the broccoli florets until tender-crisp, about 5-7 minutes.
7. Serve the coconut-crusted cod fillets with steamed broccoli.
8. Garnish with lemon wedges if desired.

Nutritional Information (per serving):

- **Calories:** 380 kcal
- **Fat:** 20g
- **Carbohydrates:** 16g
- **Protein:** 32g

<u>Herb-Roasted Chicken with Brussels Sprouts</u>

Prep Time: 15 minutes | **Cook Time:** 45 minutes | **Servings:** 4

Ingredients:

- 4 bone-in, skin-on chicken thighs
- 1-pound Brussels sprouts, trimmed and halved
- 2 tablespoons olive oil
- 3 cloves garlic, minced
- 1 teaspoon dried thyme
- 1 teaspoon dried rosemary
- 1 teaspoon dried oregano
- Salt and pepper, to taste
- Fresh parsley, for garnish (optional)

Instructions:

1. Preheat the oven to 400°F (200°C).

2. Pat the chicken thighs dry with paper towels. Place them in a large baking dish.

3. In a bowl, toss Brussels sprouts with olive oil, minced garlic, dried thyme, dried rosemary, dried oregano, salt, and pepper until evenly coated.

4. Arrange the Brussels sprouts around the chicken thighs in the baking dish.

5. Roast in the preheated oven for 40-45 minutes, or until the chicken reaches an internal temperature of 165°F (74°C) and the Brussels sprouts are tender and lightly browned.

6. Remove from the oven and let rest for a few minutes.

7. Serve the herb-roasted chicken thighs with roasted Brussels sprouts.

8. Garnish with fresh parsley if desired.

Nutritional Information (per serving):

- **Calories:** 420 kcal
- **Fat:** 25g
- **Carbohydrates:** 12g
- **Protein:** 36g

Beef and Vegetable Stew

Prep Time: 20 minutes | **Cook Time:** 2 hours | **Servings:** 6

Ingredients:

- 2 pounds beef stew meat, cubed
- 3 carrots, peeled and sliced
- 2 parsnips, peeled and sliced
- 1 celery root (celeriac), peeled and diced
- 1 onion, diced
- 3 cloves garlic, minced
- 4 cups beef broth (check for AIP compliance)
- 1 tablespoon apple cider vinegar
- 2 tablespoons coconut oil
- 1 teaspoon dried thyme
- 1 teaspoon dried rosemary
- Salt and pepper, to taste
- Fresh parsley, for garnish (optional)

Instructions:

1. In a large Dutch oven or soup pot, heat coconut oil over medium-high heat. Add cubed beef stew meat and brown on all sides, about 5-7 minutes.

2. Add diced onion, minced garlic, sliced carrots, sliced parsnips, and diced celery root to the pot with the browned beef. Sauté for 5-7 minutes until vegetables begin to soften.

3. Pour in beef broth and apple cider vinegar, stirring to deglaze the bottom of the pot.

4. Add dried thyme, dried rosemary, salt, and pepper to taste. Stir adequately to combine.

5. Bring the stew to a boil, then reduce heat to low. Cover and simmer for 1.5 to 2 hours, stirring occasionally, until the beef is tender and flavors are well combined.

6. Ladle the beef and vegetable stew into bowls.

7. Garnish with fresh parsley if desired.

Nutritional Information (per serving):

- **Calories:** 380 kcal
- **Fat:** 16g
- **Carbohydrates:** 14g
- **Protein:** 44g

Lemon-Garlic Shrimp with Zucchini Noodles

Prep Time: 15 minutes | **Cook Time:** 10 minutes | **Servings:** 4

Ingredients:

- 1-pound shrimp, peeled and deveined
- 4 medium zucchinis, spiralized into noodles
- 3 tablespoons olive oil
- 4 cloves garlic, minced
- Zest of 1 lemon
- Juice of 1 lemon
- 1/4 cup coconut milk (full-fat, canned)
- Salt and pepper, to taste
- Fresh parsley, chopped, for garnish (optional)

Instructions:

1. Heat 2 tablespoons of olive oil in a large skillet over medium-high heat. Add minced garlic and cook until fragrant, about 1 minute.

2. Add shrimp to the skillet and cook for 2-3 minutes per side, until pink and cooked through. Remove shrimp from skillet and set aside.

3. In the same skillet, add remaining 1 tablespoon of olive oil if needed. Add spiralized zucchini noodles, lemon zest, and coconut milk. Sauté for 3-4 minutes until noodles are tender but still slightly crisp.

4. Return cooked shrimp to the skillet with zucchini noodles. Add lemon juice and toss everything together until well combined.

5. Season with salt and pepper to taste.

6. Divide the lemon-garlic shrimp with zucchini noodles among serving plates.

7. Garnish with chopped fresh parsley if desired.

Nutritional Information (per serving):

- **Calories:** 290 kcal
- **Fat:** 14g
- **Carbohydrates:** 12g
- **Protein:** 30g

Pork Tenderloin with Apple Compote

Prep Time: 15 minutes | **Cook Time:** 30 minutes | **Servings:** 4

Ingredients:

For the Pork Tenderloin:

- 1 pork tenderloin (about 1 pound)
- 2 tablespoons olive oil
- Salt and pepper, to taste

For the Apple Compote:

- 2 apples, peeled, cored, and diced (AIP substitute: use compliant apples like Fuji or Honeycrisp)
- 1/2 cup apple cider (check for AIP compliance)
- 1 tablespoon coconut oil
- 1/2 teaspoon ground cinnamon
- Pinch of salt

Instructions:

1. Preheat the oven to 400°F (200°C).
2. Season the pork tenderloin generously with salt and pepper.
3. In an oven-safe skillet, heat 1 tablespoon of olive oil over medium-high heat. Sear the pork tenderloin on all sides until browned, about 2-3 minutes per side.
4. Transfer the skillet with the seared pork tenderloin to the preheated oven. Roast for 15-20 minutes, or until the internal temperature reaches 145°F (63°C). Remove from oven and let rest for 5 minutes before slicing.
5. While the pork tenderloin is roasting, prepare the apple compote.
6. In a saucepan, heat coconut oil over medium heat. Add diced apples and sauté for 3-4 minutes until they begin to soften.
7. Stir in apple cider, ground cinnamon, and a pinch of salt. Simmer for 10-12 minutes, stirring occasionally, until the apples are tender and the liquid has reduced to a thickened compote consistency.
8. Slice the pork tenderloin and serve with the warm apple compote spooned over the top.

Nutritional Information (per serving):

- **Calories:** 320 kcal
- **Fat:** 14g
- **Carbohydrates:** 18g
- **Protein:** 30g

Ginger-Turmeric Chicken Thighs with Cauliflower Rice

Prep Time: 15 minutes | **Cook Time:** 25 minutes | **Servings:** 4

Ingredients:

For the Chicken Thighs:

- 4 bone-in, skin-on chicken thighs
- 2 tablespoons olive oil
- 2 teaspoons ground ginger
- 2 teaspoons ground turmeric
- Salt and pepper, to taste

For the Cauliflower Rice:

- 1 large head cauliflower, grated into rice-like texture (or pre-riced cauliflower)
- 2 tablespoons coconut oil
- 2 cloves garlic, minced
- 1/2 teaspoon ground ginger
- Salt and pepper, to taste
- Fresh cilantro, chopped, for garnish (optional)

Instructions:

1. Preheat the oven to 400°F (200°C).

2. Rub chicken thighs with ground ginger, ground turmeric, salt, and pepper, ensuring they are well coated.

3. In an oven-safe skillet, heat olive oil over medium-high heat. Add chicken thighs, skin side down, and sear for 3-4 minutes until golden brown. Flip and sear for another 2 minutes. Transfer skillet to the preheated oven and roast for 15-20 minutes until chicken is cooked through (internal temperature of 165°F or 74°C).

4. While the chicken thighs are roasting, prepare the cauliflower rice.

5. In a large skillet, heat coconut oil over medium heat. Add minced garlic and cook for 1 minute until fragrant.

6. Add grated cauliflower, ground ginger, salt, and pepper. Sauté for 5-7 minutes until cauliflower rice is tender but still has a slight bite.

7. Divide the cauliflower rice among serving plates.

8. Place a ginger-turmeric chicken thigh on top of each plate of cauliflower rice.

9. Garnish with chopped fresh cilantro if desired.

Nutritional Information (per serving):

- **Calories:** 380 kcal
- **Fat:** 24g
- **Carbohydrates:** 10g
- **Protein:** 30g

AIP Shepherd's Pie with Ground Beef and Carrot Mash

Prep Time: 20 minutes | **Cook Time:** 40 minutes | **Servings:** 6

Ingredients:

For the Filling:

- 1 tablespoon coconut oil
- 1 onion, finely chopped
- 2 cloves garlic, minced
- 1-pound ground beef
- 2 cups carrots, peeled and diced
- 1 cup beef broth (check for AIP compliance)
- 1 tablespoon coconut aminos
- 1 teaspoon dried thyme
- Salt and pepper, to taste

For the Carrot Mash Topping:

- 4 cups carrots, peeled and chopped
- 1/4 cup coconut milk (full-fat, canned)
- 2 tablespoons coconut oil
- Salt, to taste

Instructions:

1. Place chopped carrots in a large saucepan and cover with water. Bring to a boil and cook until carrots are tender, about 10-12 minutes. Drain well.

2. Transfer cooked carrots to a food processor. Add coconut milk, coconut oil, and salt. Blend until smooth and creamy. Adjust consistency with more coconut milk if needed. Set aside.

3. Preheat oven to 400°F (200°C).

4. In a large skillet, heat coconut oil over medium heat. Add chopped onion and garlic, sauté until softened, about 3-4 minutes.

5. Add ground beef to the skillet, breaking it up with a spoon. Cook until browned and cooked through, about 5-7 minutes.

6. Add diced carrots, beef broth, coconut aminos, dried thyme, salt, and pepper to the skillet with the ground beef. Stir adequately and bring to a simmer. Cook for 10-12 minutes until carrots are tender and the liquid has reduced slightly.

7. Transfer the beef and carrot filling to a baking dish. Spread the carrot mash topping evenly over the filling.

8. Place the baking dish in the preheated oven and bake for 15-20 minutes, or until the top is lightly golden and the filling is bubbling. Next, remove from oven and let cool slightly before serving. Serve warm, garnished with fresh herbs if desired.

Nutritional Information (per serving):

- **Calories:** 320 kcal
- **Fat:** 18g
- **Carbohydrates:** 18g
- **Protein:** 22g

<u>Coconut Chicken Curry with Cauliflower Rice</u>

Prep Time: 15 minutes | **Cook Time:** 25 minutes | **Servings:** 4

Ingredients:

For the Chicken Curry:

- 1.5 pounds boneless, skinless chicken breasts, cut into cubes
- 2 tablespoons coconut oil
- 1 onion, finely chopped
- 3 cloves garlic, minced
- 1 tablespoon fresh ginger, minced
- 1 tablespoon curry powder
- 1 teaspoon ground turmeric
- 1 can (13.5 oz) coconut milk (full-fat, canned)
- 2 cups chicken broth (check for AIP compliance)
- Salt and pepper, to taste
- Fresh cilantro, chopped, for garnish (optional)

For the Cauliflower Rice:

- 1 large head cauliflower, grated into rice-like texture (or pre-riced cauliflower)
- 2 tablespoons coconut oil
- Salt and pepper, to taste

Instructions:

1. In a large skillet or pot, heat coconut oil over medium-high heat.
2. Add chopped onion, minced garlic, and minced ginger. Sauté until softened and fragrant, about 3-4 minutes.
3. Add curry powder and ground turmeric. Stir for 1 minute until spices are aromatic.
4. Add cubed chicken breasts to the skillet. Cook until chicken is browned on all sides, about 5-7 minutes.
5. Pour in coconut milk and chicken broth. Stir adequately to combine.
6. Bring to a simmer, then reduce heat to medium-low. Let it simmer uncovered for 10-15 minutes until the chicken is cooked through and the sauce has thickened slightly. Season with salt and pepper to taste.
7. While the curry is simmering, prepare the cauliflower rice. In a separate skillet, heat coconut oil over medium heat.
8. Add grated cauliflower. Season with salt and pepper. Sauté for 5-7 minutes until cauliflower rice is tender but still has a slight bite.
9. Divide the cauliflower rice among serving plates. Then spoon the coconut chicken curry over the cauliflower rice. Garnish with chopped fresh cilantro if desired.

Nutritional Information (per serving):

- **Calories:** 420 kcal
- **Fat:** 28g
- **Carbohydrates:** 12g
- **Protein:** 32g

Grilled Steak with Sautéed Spinach and Garlic

Prep Time: 10 minutes | **Cook Time:** 15 minutes | **Servings:** 4

Ingredients:

For the Steak:

- 4 beef sirloin steaks, about 6 oz each
- Salt and freshly ground black pepper, to taste
- 2 tablespoons olive oil

For the Sautéed Spinach and Garlic:

- 2 tablespoons olive oil
- 4 cloves garlic, minced
- 10 oz fresh spinach leaves, washed and dried
- Salt and freshly ground black pepper, to taste
- Lemon wedges, for serving (optional)

Instructions:

1. Preheat the grill to medium-high heat.
2. Season the steaks generously with salt and pepper on both sides.
3. Brush each steak with olive oil.
4. Place the steaks on the preheated grill. Grill for about 4-5 minutes per side for medium-rare, or adjust cooking time according to desired doneness.
5. Take out the steaks from the grill and let them rest for 5 minutes before slicing.
6. While the steaks are resting, heat 2 tablespoons of olive oil in a large skillet over medium heat.
7. Add minced garlic and sauté for about 1 minute until fragrant.
8. Add the fresh spinach leaves to the skillet in batches, tossing gently until wilted.
9. Season with salt and pepper to taste.
10. Divide the sautéed spinach among serving plates.
11. Slice the grilled steaks against the grain and place them on top of the spinach.
12. Serve with lemon wedges if desired.

Nutritional Information (per serving):

- **Calories:** 420 kcal
- **Fat:** 26g
- **Carbohydrates:** 4g
- **Protein:** 42g

Snacks Recipes

Apple Slices with Coconut Butter

Prep Time: 10 minutes | **Cook Time:** 0 minutes | **Servings:** 2

Ingredients:

- 2 medium apples, cored and sliced
- 2 tablespoons coconut butter, softened
- Optional: Cinnamon powder for sprinkling

Instructions:

1. Wash and core the apples. Slice them into thin rounds or wedges.
2. Spread the softened coconut butter evenly over the apple slices.
3. Optionally, sprinkle cinnamon powder over the coated apple slices.
4. Serve immediately or refrigerate for a chilled treat.

Nutritional Information (per serving):

- **Calories:** 120 kcal
- **Fat:** 7g
- **Carbohydrates:** 16g
- **Protein:** 1g

Plantain Chips with Guacamole

Prep Time: 15 minutes | **Cook Time:** 15 minutes | **Servings:** 2

Ingredients:

- 2 green plantains
- 2 tablespoons coconut oil, melted
- Salt, to taste
- 1 ripe avocado
- 1 tablespoon fresh lime juice
- 1 small garlic clove, minced
- 1 tablespoon chopped fresh cilantro (optional)

Instructions:

1. Preheat the oven to 375°F (190°C). Line a baking sheet with parchment paper.
2. Peel the plantains and slice them thinly using a mandoline slicer or knife. Place the plantain slices in a bowl.
3. Drizzle melted coconut oil over the plantain slices and toss to coat evenly. Arrange the slices in a single layer on the prepared baking sheet. Sprinkle with salt.
4. Bake in the preheated oven for 10-15 minutes, flipping halfway through, until the plantain chips are golden and crispy. Remove from oven and let cool slightly.
5. While the plantain chips are baking, prepare the guacamole. Mash the avocado in a bowl until smooth. Add lime juice, minced garlic, and chopped cilantro (if using). Mix adequately to combine.
6. Serve the plantain chips with the guacamole.

Nutritional Information (per serving):

- **Calories:** 280 kcal
- **Fat:** 19g
- **Carbohydrates:** 30g
- **Protein:** 3g

Carrot and Celery Sticks with AIP Ranch Dip

Prep Time: 15 minutes | **Cook Time:** 0 minutes | **Servings:** 2

Ingredients:

- 2 medium carrots, peeled and cut into sticks
- 2 celery stalks, cut into sticks
- *For AIP Ranch Dip:*
  - 1/2 cup coconut milk (full-fat, canned)
  - 1 tablespoon fresh lemon juice
  - 1/2 teaspoon dried parsley
  - 1/2 teaspoon dried dill
  - 1/4 teaspoon garlic powder (use garlic-infused oil for AIP)
  - Salt, to taste

Instructions:

1. Prepare the carrots and celery by peeling and cutting them into stick shapes. Place them in a serving dish.
2. In a small bowl, combine the coconut milk, fresh lemon juice, dried parsley, dried dill, garlic powder (or garlic-infused oil), and salt. Mix adequately until all ingredients are thoroughly combined.
3. Adjust the seasoning to taste, adding more salt or lemon juice if desired.
4. Serve the carrot and celery sticks alongside the AIP Ranch Dip.

Nutritional Information (per serving):

- **Calories:** 150 kcal
- **Fat:** 13g
- **Carbohydrates:** 8g
- **Protein:** 2g

AIP Beef Jerky

Prep Time: 20 minutes | **Cook Time:** 4-6 hours (drying time) | **Servings:** 4

Ingredients:

- 1-pound lean beef (such as top round or sirloin), thinly sliced against the grain
- 1/4 cup coconut aminos
- 2 tablespoons apple cider vinegar
- 1 tablespoon olive oil
- 1/2 teaspoon garlic powder (use garlic-infused oil for AIP)
- 1/2 teaspoon onion powder
- 1/2 teaspoon dried oregano
- 1/4 teaspoon ground ginger
- Salt, to taste

Instructions:

1. In a bowl, combine coconut aminos, apple cider vinegar, olive oil, garlic powder (or garlic-infused oil), onion powder, dried oregano, ground ginger, and salt. Mix adequately to create the marinade.

2. Place the thinly sliced beef into a resealable plastic bag or shallow dish. Pour the marinade over the beef, ensuring all pieces are coated. Seal the bag or cover the dish and refrigerate for at least 4 hours, preferably overnight.

3. Preheat your oven to 175°F (80°C) or the lowest setting.

4. Take out the marinated beef from the refrigerator and drain off any excess marinade. Pat the beef slices dry with paper towels.

5. Arrange the beef slices on wire racks placed over baking sheets or directly on baking sheets lined with parchment paper.

6. Place the beef in the preheated oven and bake for 4-6 hours, or until the jerky is dried and firm, flipping the slices halfway through the drying process.

7. Once dried to your desired texture, take out the beef jerky from the oven and let it cool completely before storing in an airtight container.

Nutritional Information (per serving):

- **Calories:** 180 kcal
- **Fat:** 7g
- **Carbohydrates:** 5g
- **Protein:** 22g

Mixed Berry Fruit Leather

Prep Time: 15 minutes | **Cook Time:** 4-6 hours (drying time) | **Servings:** 4

Ingredients:

- 2 cups mixed berries (such as strawberries, blueberries, raspberries), fresh or frozen
- 1 tablespoon fresh lemon juice
- 1 tablespoon honey (optional, omit for strict AIP)
- Optional: 1/4 teaspoon ground cinnamon

Instructions:

1. Preheat your oven to the lowest setting, typically around 140°F (60°C).
2. If using fresh berries, rinse them thoroughly. If using frozen berries, thaw them and drain any excess liquid.
3. In a blender or food processor, combine the mixed berries, fresh lemon juice, honey (if using), and ground cinnamon (if using). Blend until smooth.
4. Line a baking sheet with parchment paper. Pour the berry mixture onto the parchment paper and spread it evenly into a thin layer, about 1/8 inch thick.
5. Place the baking sheet in the preheated oven and bake for 4-6 hours, or until the fruit leather is dried and no longer sticky to the touch. Rotate the baking sheet halfway through the drying process for even drying.
6. Once dried, take out the fruit leather from the oven and let it cool completely.
7. Using kitchen scissors or a knife, cut the fruit leather into strips or shapes. Roll the strips with parchment paper or store them in an airtight container.

Nutritional Information (per serving):

- **Calories:** 60 kcal
- **Fat:** 0.5g
- **Carbohydrates:** 15g
- **Protein:** 1g

Coconut Macaroons

Prep Time: 15 minutes | **Cook Time:** 20 minutes | **Servings:** 12

Ingredients:

- 2 cups shredded coconut (unsweetened)
- 1/2 cup coconut milk (full-fat, canned)
- 1/4 cup honey (optional, omit for strict AIP)
- 1 teaspoon vanilla extract (AIP-compliant)
- Pinch of salt

Instructions:

1. Preheat your oven to 325°F (165°C). Line a baking sheet with parchment paper.

2. In a mixing bowl, combine shredded coconut, coconut milk, honey (if using), vanilla extract, and a pinch of salt. Mix until the ingredients are well combined and the coconut is fully coated.

3. Using a tablespoon or cookie scoop, scoop the mixture into small mounds and place them onto the prepared baking sheet, spacing them about 1 inch apart.

4. Bake in the preheated oven for 18-20 minutes, or until the macaroons are golden brown on the edges.

5. Remove from the oven and let the macaroons cool on the baking sheet for a few minutes before transferring them to a wire rack to cool completely.

Nutritional Information (per serving):

- **Calories:** 120 kcal
- **Fat:** 10g
- **Carbohydrates:** 8g
- **Protein:** 1g

Baked Kale Chips

Prep Time: 10 minutes | **Cook Time:** 15 minutes | **Servings:** 2

Ingredients:

- 1 bunch of kale, washed and thoroughly dried
- 1 tablespoon olive oil
- Salt, to taste

Instructions:

1. Preheat your oven to 300°F (150°C). Line a baking sheet with parchment paper.
2. Take out the kale leaves from the thick stems and tear them into bite-sized pieces. Ensure the kale is completely dry.
3. In a large bowl, drizzle the kale pieces with olive oil and sprinkle with salt. Toss to coat evenly.
4. Spread the kale pieces in a single layer on the prepared baking sheet.
5. Bake in the preheated oven for 15 minutes, or until the edges are crispy but not burnt. Check halfway through and turn the leaves if necessary.
6. Remove from the oven and let cool on the baking sheet for a few minutes before serving.

Nutritional Information (per serving):

- **Calories:** 50 kcal
- **Fat:** 3.5g
- **Carbohydrates:** 5g
- **Protein:** 2g

Avocado and Tuna Boats

Prep Time: 10 minutes | **Cook Time:** 0 minutes | **Servings:** 2

Ingredients:

- 2 ripe avocados, halved and pitted
- 1 can (5 ounces) tuna, packed in water, drained
- 1 tablespoon olive oil
- 1 tablespoon fresh lemon juice
- 1 tablespoon chopped fresh parsley (optional)
- Salt, to taste

Instructions:

1. In a small bowl, combine the drained tuna, olive oil, fresh lemon juice, chopped fresh parsley (if using), and salt. Mix adequately.

2. Using a spoon, scoop a small amount of avocado flesh from each avocado half to create a slightly larger cavity for the tuna mixture.

3. Fill each avocado half with the tuna mixture, distributing it evenly.

4. Serve immediately.

Nutritional Information (per serving):

- **Calories:** 300 kcal
- **Fat:** 22g
- **Carbohydrates:** 12g
- **Protein:** 16g

AIP Granola Bars with Coconut and Dried Fruit

Prep Time: 15 minutes | **Cook Time:** 25 minutes | **Servings:** 8

Ingredients:

- 1 cup shredded coconut (unsweetened)
- 1/2 cup dried fruit (such as blueberries, cranberries, or apricots), diced
- 1/4 cup coconut oil
- 1/4 cup honey (optional, omit for strict AIP)
- 1 teaspoon vanilla extract (AIP-compliant)
- Pinch of salt

Instructions:

1. Preheat your oven to 325°F (165°C). Line an 8x8 inch baking dish with parchment paper.
2. In a large mixing bowl, combine shredded coconut and diced dried fruit.
3. In a small saucepan over low heat, melt the coconut oil. Remove from heat and stir in honey (if using), vanilla extract, and a pinch of salt.
4. Pour the coconut oil mixture over the coconut and dried fruit mixture. Stir adequately to combine, ensuring the dry ingredients are well coated.
5. Press the mixture firmly and evenly into the prepared baking dish.
6. Bake in the preheated oven for 20-25 minutes, or until the edges are golden brown.
7. Remove from the oven and let cool completely in the baking dish.
8. Once cooled, lift the granola out of the baking dish using the parchment paper and cut it into bars.

Nutritional Information (per serving):

- **Calories:** 180 kcal
- **Fat:** 14g
- **Carbohydrates:** 15g
- **Protein:** 1g

Cucumber Slices with Smoked Salmon

Prep Time: 10 minutes | **Cook Time:** 0 minutes | **Servings:** 4

Ingredients:

- 1 large cucumber, sliced into rounds
- 4 ounces smoked salmon, cut into small pieces
- 1 tablespoon fresh lemon juice
- 1 tablespoon fresh dill, chopped (optional)
- Salt, to taste

Instructions:

1. Arrange the cucumber rounds on a serving platter.
2. Place a small piece of smoked salmon on top of each cucumber slice.
3. Drizzle the fresh lemon juice over the smoked salmon and cucumber slices.
4. Sprinkle with chopped fresh dill (if using) and salt to taste.
5. Serve immediately.

Nutritional Information (per serving):

- **Calories:** 70 kcal
- **Fat:** 4g
- **Carbohydrates:** 2g
- **Protein:** 6g

Mango and Pineapple Smoothie

Prep Time: 10 minutes | **Cook Time:** 0 minutes | **Servings:** 2

Ingredients:

- 1 cup fresh mango, diced

- 1 cup fresh pineapple, diced

- 1 cup coconut milk

- 1 tablespoon fresh lime juice

- 1 teaspoon fresh ginger, grated (optional)

Instructions:

1. In a blender, combine the diced fresh mango, diced fresh pineapple, coconut milk, fresh lime juice, and grated fresh ginger (if using).

2. Blend until smooth and creamy.

3. Pour into glasses and serve immediately.

Nutritional Information (per serving):

- **Calories:** 150 kcal

- **Fat:** 7g

- **Carbohydrates:** 23g

- **Protein:** 1g

<u>Coconut Milk Popsicles with Berries</u>

Prep Time: 10 minutes | **Cook Time:** 0 minutes | **Servings:** 6

Ingredients:

- 1 can (13.5 ounces) full-fat coconut milk
- 1 tablespoon honey (optional, for sweetness)
- 1 teaspoon vanilla extract (optional)
- 1 cup mixed berries, fresh or frozen

Instructions:

1. In a bowl, whisk together the full-fat coconut milk, honey (if using), and vanilla extract (if using) until well combined.
2. Divide the mixed berries (fresh or frozen) evenly among popsicle molds.
3. Pour the coconut milk mixture over the berries in the molds, filling each mold to the top.
4. Insert popsicle sticks and freeze for at least 4 hours or until solid.
5. To take out the popsicles from the molds, run warm water over the outside of the molds for a few seconds.

Nutritional Information (per serving):

- **Calories:** 130 kcal
- **Fat:** 10g
- **Carbohydrates:** 9g
- **Protein:** 1g

Chapter 5: Maintenance Phase Recipes

Breakfast Recipes

Sweet Potato and Kale Breakfast Hash

Prep Time: 15 minutes | **Cook Time:** 25 minutes | **Number of Servings:** 4

Ingredients:

- 2 medium sweet potatoes, peeled and diced
- 2 tablespoons olive oil
- 1 medium onion, diced
- 2 cloves garlic, minced
- 1 red bell pepper, diced
- 1-pound ground turkey
- 1 teaspoon dried oregano
- 1 teaspoon dried thyme
- 1/2 teaspoon sea salt
- 1/4 teaspoon ground black pepper
- 4 cups kale, chopped
- 1 avocado, sliced (optional for serving)

Instructions:

1. Heat 1 tablespoon of olive oil in a large skillet over medium heat. Add the diced sweet potatoes and cook for about 10 minutes, stirring occasionally, until they start to soften.

2. Push the sweet potatoes to the side of the skillet and add the remaining 1 tablespoon of olive oil. Add the diced onion and minced garlic. Sauté for 2-3 minutes until fragrant.

3. Add the diced red bell pepper to the skillet and cook for an additional 5 minutes until all vegetables are tender.

4. Push the vegetables to the side of the skillet and add the ground turkey. Cook, breaking it apart with a spatula, until no longer pink, about 6-8 minutes.

5. Stir in the dried oregano, dried thyme, sea salt, and ground black pepper.

6. Add the chopped kale to the skillet and cook for 2-3 minutes until wilted.

7. Mix all ingredients together until well combined. Adjust seasoning to taste.

8. Serve hot, optionally topped with sliced avocado.

Nutritional Information (per serving):

- **Calories:** 320 kcal
- **Fat:** 18 grams (g)
- **Carbohydrates:** 22 grams (g)
- **Protein:** 21 grams (g)

<u>Zucchini and Bacon Fritters with Avocado</u>

Prep Time: 15 minutes | **Cook Time:** 20 minutes | **Number of Servings:** 4

Ingredients:

- 2 medium zucchinis, grated
- 1 teaspoon sea salt
- 4 slices bacon, cooked and crumbled
- 1/4 cup coconut flour
- 2 large eggs, beaten
- 1/4 cup green onions, finely chopped
- 2 cloves garlic, minced
- 2 tablespoons olive oil
- 1 avocado, sliced (for serving)

Instructions:

1. Place the grated zucchini in a colander and sprinkle with sea salt. Let it sit for 10 minutes, then squeeze out the excess moisture using a clean towel.

2. In a large bowl, combine the drained zucchini, crumbled bacon, coconut flour, beaten eggs, finely chopped green onions, and minced garlic. Mix adequately.

3. Heat 1 tablespoon of olive oil in a large skillet over medium heat.

4. Scoop about 1/4 cup of the zucchini mixture and shape into a patty. Place it in the skillet. Repeat with the remaining mixture, cooking 4-5 fritters at a time.

5. Cook the fritters for 3-4 minutes on each side until golden brown and crispy.

6. Take out the fritters from the skillet and place them on a paper towel-lined plate to drain any excess oil. Repeat with the remaining mixture, adding more olive oil to the skillet as needed.

7. Serve the fritters hot, topped with sliced avocado.

Nutritional Information (per serving):

- **Calories:** 290 kcal
- **Fat:** 19 grams (g)
- **Carbohydrates:** 11 grams (g)
- **Protein:** 16 grams (g)

Coconut Yogurt Parfait with Berries and Honey

Prep Time: 10 minutes | **Cook Time:** 0 minutes | **Number of Servings:** 4

Ingredients:

- 2 cups coconut yogurt
- 1 cup mixed berries (blueberries, raspberries, strawberries), sliced
- 2 tablespoons raw honey
- 1/4 cup unsweetened shredded coconut
- 1/4 cup chopped nuts (almonds, walnuts) (optional, if reintroduced successfully)

Instructions:

1. In a small bowl, mix the coconut yogurt until smooth.

2. Layer 1/2 cup of coconut yogurt into the bottom of each of four serving glasses.

3. Add a layer of mixed sliced berries on top of the yogurt in each glass.

4. Drizzle 1/2 tablespoon of raw honey over the berries in each glass.

5. Sprinkle 1 tablespoon of unsweetened shredded coconut on top of the honey in each glass.

6. If using chopped nuts, sprinkle 1 tablespoon of chopped nuts over the shredded coconut in each glass.

7. Repeat the layers if there is remaining yogurt, berries, honey, shredded coconut, and nuts.

8. Serve immediately, or chill in the refrigerator for up to 2 hours before serving.

Nutritional Information (per serving):

- **Calories:** 210 kcal
- **Fat:** 13 grams (g)
- **Carbohydrates:** 18 grams (g)
- **Protein:** 5 grams (g)

Scrambled Eggs with Spinach and Mushrooms

Prep Time: 10 minutes | **Cook Time:** 10 minutes | **Number of Servings:** 2

Ingredients:

- 4 large eggs
- 1 tablespoon olive oil
- 1 cup spinach leaves, chopped
- 1 cup mushrooms, sliced
- 1/4 teaspoon sea salt
- 1/4 teaspoon ground black pepper
- Fresh herbs (such as parsley or chives) for garnish (optional)

Instructions:

1. Crack the eggs into a bowl and whisk until well combined.
2. Heat olive oil in a non-stick skillet over medium heat.
3. Add the sliced mushrooms to the skillet and cook for 3-4 minutes until they start to soften.
4. Add the chopped spinach to the skillet and cook for another 2 minutes until wilted.
5. Season the vegetables with sea salt and ground black pepper.
6. Pour the whisked eggs into the skillet over the vegetables. Let the eggs sit for a few seconds until they start to set on the bottom.
7. Gently stir the eggs and vegetables together with a spatula, continuing to cook until the eggs are fully scrambled and cooked to your desired consistency.
8. Remove from heat and garnish with fresh herbs if desired.

Nutritional Information (per serving):

- **Calories:** 220 kcal
- **Fat:** 15 grams (g)
- **Carbohydrates:** 4 grams (g)
- **Protein:** 16 grams (g)

Banana and Flaxseed Smoothie

Prep Time: 5 minutes | **Cook Time:** 0 minutes | **Number of Servings:** 2

Ingredients:

- 2 ripe bananas, peeled and sliced
- 1 cup unsweetened almond milk
- 2 tablespoons ground flaxseed
- 1 tablespoon almond butter
- 1/2 teaspoon ground cinnamon
- Ice cubes (optional)

Instructions:

1. In a blender, combine the sliced bananas, unsweetened almond milk, ground flaxseed, almond butter, and ground cinnamon.
2. Blend until smooth and creamy, adding ice cubes if desired for a colder smoothie.
3. Pour into glasses and serve immediately.

Nutritional Information (per serving):

- **Calories:** 220 kcal
- **Fat:** 10 grams (g)
- **Carbohydrates:** 30 grams (g)
- **Protein:** 5 grams (g)

Chia Seed Pudding with Mango and Coconut

Prep Time: 5 minutes | **Cook Time:** 0 minutes | **Chill Time:** 2 hours | **Number of Servings:** 2

Ingredients:

- 1/4 cup chia seeds

- 1 cup unsweetened coconut milk

- 1 tablespoon raw honey or maple syrup (optional, for sweetness)

- 1 ripe mango, peeled and diced

- 2 tablespoons unsweetened shredded coconut

Instructions:

1. In a mixing bowl, combine the chia seeds and unsweetened coconut milk. Stir adequately to mix thoroughly.

2. If using, add raw honey or maple syrup for sweetness and stir until fully incorporated.

3. Cover the bowl and refrigerate for at least 2 hours or overnight, allowing the chia seeds to absorb the liquid and thicken into a pudding-like consistency.

4. Before serving, stir the chia seed pudding mixture to ensure it's well combined and smooth.

5. Divide the pudding into serving dishes.

6. Top each serving with diced mango and sprinkle with unsweetened shredded coconut.

Nutritional Information (per serving):

- **Calories:** 250 kcal

- **Fat:** 15 grams (g)

- **Carbohydrates:** 25 grams (g)

- **Protein:** 6 grams (g)

AIP Pancakes with Maple Syrup and Blueberries

Prep Time: 10 minutes | **Cook Time:** 10 minutes | **Number of Servings:** 2-3

Ingredients:

- 1 cup mashed sweet potatoes (about 2 medium sweet potatoes, cooked and mashed)
- 2 tablespoons coconut flour
- 2 tablespoons arrowroot flour
- 2 tablespoons coconut oil, melted
- 2 tablespoons coconut milk (unsweetened)
- 1 teaspoon vanilla extract
- 1/2 teaspoon baking soda
- 1/4 teaspoon sea salt
- Coconut oil or ghee for cooking
- Maple syrup and fresh blueberries for serving

Instructions:

1. In a mixing bowl, combine the mashed sweet potatoes, coconut flour, arrowroot flour, melted coconut oil, coconut milk, vanilla extract, baking soda, and sea salt. Mix adequately until smooth and thoroughly combined.

2. Heat a skillet or griddle over medium heat and lightly grease with coconut oil or ghee.

3. Pour about 1/4 cup of batter onto the skillet for each pancake. Spread slightly with a spoon to form a round shape.

4. Cook for about 3-4 minutes on one side, until bubbles start to form on the surface of the pancake and the edges begin to set.

5. Carefully flip the pancake and cook for another 2-3 minutes on the other side, until golden brown and cooked through.

6. Repeat with the remaining batter, adding more coconut oil or ghee to the skillet as needed.

7. Serve the pancakes warm, topped with maple syrup and fresh blueberries.

Nutritional Information (per serving):

- **Calories:** 280 kcal
- **Fat:** 14 grams (g)
- **Carbohydrates:** 35 grams (g)
- **Protein:** 5 grams (g)

Breakfast Sausage Patties with Sweet Potato Mash

Prep Time: 15 minutes | **Cook Time:** 25 minutes | **Number of Servings:** 4

Ingredients:

- 1-pound ground turkey or chicken
- 1 teaspoon dried sage
- 1/2 teaspoon dried thyme
- 1/2 teaspoon garlic powder
- 1/2 teaspoon onion powder
- 1/2 teaspoon sea salt
- 1/4 teaspoon ground black pepper
- 2 tablespoons olive oil, divided
- 2 medium sweet potatoes, peeled and diced
- 1/4 cup coconut milk (unsweetened)

Instructions:

1. In a mixing bowl, combine the ground turkey or chicken with dried sage, dried thyme, garlic powder, onion powder, sea salt, and ground black pepper. Mix adequately until all the spices are evenly distributed.

2. Shape the seasoned meat mixture into small patties.

3. Heat 1 tablespoon of olive oil in a skillet over medium heat. Cook the sausage patties for about 5-6 minutes on each side, or until fully cooked through and browned. Remove from the skillet and set aside.

4. In the same skillet, add the remaining 1 tablespoon of olive oil and heat over medium heat. Add the diced sweet potatoes and cook for about 10-12 minutes, or until tender and lightly browned, stirring occasionally.

5. Once the sweet potatoes are cooked, mash them with a fork or potato masher until smooth.

6. Stir in the coconut milk until well combined and heated through.

7. Serve the breakfast sausage patties alongside the sweet potato mash.

Nutritional Information (per serving):

- **Calories:** 350 kcal
- **Fat:** 18 grams (g)
- **Carbohydrates:** 20 grams (g)
- **Protein:** 25 grams (g)

<u>Avocado Toast on AIP Bread with Poached Eggs</u>

Prep Time: 15 minutes | **Cook Time:** 10 minutes | **Number of Servings:** 2

Ingredients:

- 4 slices AIP-friendly bread (such as cassava flour bread or coconut flour bread)
- 1 ripe avocado
- Juice of 1/2 lemon
- Sea salt and ground black pepper, to taste
- 4 large eggs
- Fresh chives or parsley, chopped, for garnish (optional)

Instructions:

1. Toast the AIP-friendly bread slices until they are golden brown and crispy.

2. While the bread is toasting, prepare the avocado spread: Scoop the flesh of the avocado into a bowl, add the lemon juice, sea salt, and ground black pepper. Mash together until smooth and well combined.

3. Poach the eggs: Bring a large pot of water to a gentle simmer. Crack each egg into a small bowl or cup. Carefully slide each egg into the simmering water and cook for about 3-4 minutes until the whites are set but the yolks are still runny.

4. Take out the poached eggs with a slotted spoon and drain on a paper towel.

5. Spread the mashed avocado evenly onto each slice of toasted bread.

6. Carefully place a poached egg on top of each slice of avocado toast.

7. Garnish with chopped fresh chives or parsley, if desired.

8. Serve immediately while the eggs are still warm.

Nutritional Information (per serving):

- **Calories:** 320 kcal
- **Fat:** 18 grams (g)
- **Carbohydrates:** 25 grams (g)
- **Protein:** 15 grams (g)

Mixed Berry Smoothie Bowl with Hemp Seeds

Prep Time: 10 minutes | **Cook Time:** 0 minutes | **Number of Servings:** 2

Ingredients:

- 1 cup mixed berries (such as strawberries, blueberries, raspberries)
- 1 ripe banana, peeled and sliced
- 1/2 cup unsweetened almond milk
- 2 tablespoons hemp seeds
- 1 tablespoon raw honey or maple syrup (optional, for sweetness)
- Fresh berries, sliced banana, and shredded coconut for topping (optional)

Instructions:

1. In a blender, combine the mixed berries, sliced banana, unsweetened almond milk, and hemp seeds.
2. If using, add raw honey or maple syrup for sweetness.
3. Blend until smooth and creamy, adding more almond milk if needed to reach desired consistency.
4. Pour the smoothie into bowls.
5. Top with fresh berries, sliced banana, and shredded coconut if desired.
6. Serve immediately.

Nutritional Information (per serving):

- **Calories:** 250 kcal
- **Fat:** 10 grams (g)
- **Carbohydrates:** 35 grams (g)
- **Protein:** 8 grams (g)

Butternut Squash and Apple Hash

Prep Time: 15 minutes | **Cook Time:** 20 minutes | **Number of Servings:** 4

Ingredients:

- 1 small butternut squash, peeled, seeded, and diced
- 2 apples, cored and diced (use sweet varieties like Gala or Fuji)
- 1 onion, diced
- 2 tablespoons olive oil
- 1 teaspoon ground cinnamon
- 1/2 teaspoon ground nutmeg
- Sea salt and freshly ground black pepper, to taste
- Fresh parsley, chopped, for garnish (optional)

Instructions:

1. Heat olive oil in a large skillet over medium heat.
2. Add the diced butternut squash to the skillet and cook for about 8-10 minutes, stirring occasionally, until it starts to soften.
3. Add the diced apples and onion to the skillet with the butternut squash. Cook for another 8-10 minutes, or until the squash and apples are tender and lightly browned.
4. Season the hash with ground cinnamon, ground nutmeg, sea salt, and freshly ground black pepper. Stir adequately to combine and cook for another minute to let the flavors meld.
5. Remove from heat and garnish with chopped fresh parsley if desired.
6. Serve warm as a side dish or main course.

Nutritional Information (per serving):

- **Calories:** 180 kcal
- **Fat:** 7 grams (g)
- **Carbohydrates:** 30 grams (g)
- **Protein:** 2 grams (g)

Smoked Salmon and Dill Omelette

Prep Time: 10 minutes | **Cook Time:** 10 minutes | **Number of Servings:** 2

Ingredients:

- 4 large eggs
- 2 ounces smoked salmon, chopped
- 1 tablespoon fresh dill, chopped
- 1/4 cup unsweetened almond milk
- Sea salt and ground black pepper, to taste
- 1 tablespoon ghee or coconut oil

Instructions:

1. In a bowl, whisk together the eggs and unsweetened almond milk until well combined.
2. Stir in the chopped smoked salmon and fresh dill into the egg mixture.
3. Season with sea salt and ground black pepper to taste.
4. Heat ghee or coconut oil in a non-stick skillet over medium heat.
5. Pour the egg mixture into the skillet and let it cook for 2-3 minutes, or until the edges start to set.
6. Using a spatula, gently lift the edges of the omelette and tilt the skillet to let the uncooked egg flow underneath.
7. Continue cooking for another 2-3 minutes, or until the omelette is mostly set but still slightly runny on top.
8. Carefully fold the omelette in half with the spatula and cook for another 1-2 minutes until fully set and lightly golden.
9. Slide the omelette onto a plate and garnish with additional fresh dill if desired.
10. Serve immediately.

Nutritional Information (per serving):

- **Calories:** 280 kcal
- **Fat:** 20 grams (g)
- **Carbohydrates:** 2 grams (g)
- **Protein:** 22 grams (g)

Lunch Recipes

Grilled Chicken Salad with Mixed Greens and Avocado

Prep Time: 15 minutes | **Cook Time:** 15 minutes | **Number of Servings:** 4

Ingredients:

- 1-pound chicken breasts, boneless and skinless
- 8 cups mixed salad greens
- 2 avocados, sliced
- 1 cucumber, sliced
- 1 cup cherry tomatoes, halved
- 1/4 cup red onion, thinly sliced
- 1/4 cup fresh cilantro leaves
- Juice of 1 lemon
- 2 tablespoons olive oil
- Salt and pepper to taste

Instructions:

1. Preheat grill to medium-high heat.

2. Season chicken breasts with salt and pepper.

3. Grill chicken for about 6-7 minutes per side, or until fully cooked (internal temperature of 165°F or 74°C). Remove from grill and let rest for 5 minutes before slicing.

4. In a large bowl, combine mixed greens, avocado slices, cucumber slices, cherry tomatoes, red onion slices, and cilantro leaves.

5. In a small bowl, whisk together lemon juice, olive oil, salt, and pepper.

6. Drizzle dressing over the salad and toss gently to combine.

7. Slice grilled chicken breasts and place them on top of the salad.

8. Serve immediately.

Nutritional Information (per serving):

- **Calories:** 350 kcal
- **Fat:** 20g
- **Carbohydrates:** 12g
- **Proteins:** 30g

Turkey and Cranberry Lettuce Wraps

Prep Time: 15 minutes | **Cook Time:** 10 minutes | **Number of Servings:** 4

Ingredients:

- 1-pound ground turkey
- 1 tablespoon olive oil
- 1/2 cup onion, finely diced
- 2 cloves garlic, minced
- 1 teaspoon dried thyme
- 1/2 teaspoon dried sage
- Salt and pepper to taste
- 1/4 cup dried cranberries
- 1/4 cup chopped pecans
- 1/4 cup fresh parsley, chopped
- 8 large lettuce leaves (such as iceberg or butter lettuce)

Instructions:

1. Heat olive oil in a large skillet over medium heat.
2. Add diced onion and cook until translucent, about 3-4 minutes.
3. Add minced garlic and cook for 1 minute until fragrant.
4. Add ground turkey to the skillet, breaking it apart with a spoon, and cook until browned and cooked through, about 6-7 minutes.
5. Stir in dried thyme, dried sage, salt, and pepper.
6. Add dried cranberries and chopped pecans to the skillet, stirring to combine, and cook for another 1-2 minutes.
7. Remove from heat and stir in chopped fresh parsley.
8. To assemble, place a spoonful of the turkey mixture onto each lettuce leaf.
9. Roll up and secure with toothpicks if needed.

Nutritional Information (per serving):

- **Calories:** 300 kcal
- **Fat:** 15g
- **Carbohydrates:** 10g
- **Proteins:** 30g

Shrimp and Mango Salad with Lime Vinaigrette

Prep Time: 20 minutes | **Cook Time:** 5 minutes | **Number of Servings:** 4

Ingredients:

- 1-pound shrimp, peeled and deveined
- 2 mangos, peeled and diced
- 1 red bell pepper, diced
- 1/2 red onion, thinly sliced
- 1/4 cup fresh cilantro leaves, chopped
- 1/4 cup fresh mint leaves, chopped
- Juice of 2 limes
- 3 tablespoons olive oil
- Salt and pepper to taste
- Mixed salad greens for serving

Instructions:

1. Bring a pot of water to boil. Add shrimp and cook for 2-3 minutes until shrimp are pink and opaque. Drain and rinse under cold water to stop cooking. Set aside.

2. In a large bowl, combine diced mango, diced red bell pepper, thinly sliced red onion, chopped cilantro leaves, and chopped mint leaves.

3. Add cooked shrimp to the bowl.

4. In a small bowl, whisk together lime juice, olive oil, salt, and pepper to make the vinaigrette.

5. Pour the vinaigrette over the shrimp and mango mixture in the large bowl. Toss gently to combine.

6. To serve, divide mixed salad greens among plates and top with the shrimp and mango mixture.

Nutritional Information (per serving):

- **Calories:** 250 kcal
- **Fat:** 10g
- **Carbohydrates:** 20g
- **Proteins:** 25g

<u>Beef and Broccoli Stir-fry with Coconut Aminos</u>

Prep Time: 15 minutes | **Cook Time:** 15 minutes | **Number of Servings:** 4

Ingredients:

- 1-pound flank steak, thinly sliced against the grain
- 1 tablespoon olive oil
- 2 cups broccoli florets
- 1 red bell pepper, thinly sliced
- 1/2 cup sliced mushrooms
- 3 cloves garlic, minced
- 1-inch piece of ginger, grated
- 1/4 cup coconut aminos
- 2 tablespoons apple cider vinegar
- Salt and pepper to taste
- Sesame seeds for garnish (optional)

Instructions:

1. Heat olive oil in a large skillet or wok over medium-high heat.

2. Add sliced flank steak to the skillet and stir-fry for 2-3 minutes until browned. Remove from skillet and set aside.

3. In the same skillet, add broccoli florets, red bell pepper slices, and sliced mushrooms. Stir-fry for about 3-4 minutes until vegetables are tender-crisp.

4. Add minced garlic and grated ginger to the skillet, stirring constantly for about 1 minute until fragrant.

5. Return the cooked flank steak to the skillet.

6. Pour coconut aminos and apple cider vinegar over the beef and vegetables. Stir adequately to combine and coat everything evenly.

7. Cook for another 1-2 minutes until everything is heated through.

8. Season with salt and pepper to taste.

9. To serve, sprinkle with sesame seeds if desired.

Nutritional Information (per serving):

- **Calories:** 300 kcal
- **Fat:** 15g
- **Carbohydrates:** 10g
- **Proteins:** 30g

AIP Caesar Salad with Homemade Dressing and Anchovies

Prep Time: 15 minutes | **Cook Time:** 0 minutes | **Number of Servings:** 4

Ingredients:

- For the Dressing:
    - 1/2 cup avocado mayo
    - 2 cloves garlic, minced
    - 1 tablespoon nutritional yeast
    - 1 tablespoon lemon juice
    - 1 teaspoon apple cider vinegar
    - Salt and pepper to taste

- For the Salad:
    - 1 large head of romaine lettuce, chopped
    - 1/4 cup sliced cucumber
    - 1/4 cup sliced radishes
    - 1/4 cup chopped green onions
    - 1/4 cup chopped fresh parsley
    - 4-6 anchovy fillets, chopped (optional)
    - 1/4 cup chopped cooked chicken (optional, for added protein)

Instructions:

1. Prepare the Dressing: In a small bowl, combine avocado mayo, minced garlic, nutritional yeast, lemon juice, apple cider vinegar, salt, and pepper. Whisk until smooth and well combined.

2. Assemble the Salad: In a large bowl, combine chopped romaine lettuce, sliced cucumber, sliced radishes, chopped green onions, and chopped fresh parsley.

3. Add the Anchovies: If using, add chopped anchovy fillets to the salad.

4. Add Protein (Optional): If desired, add chopped cooked chicken for additional protein.

5. Pour the Dressing: Drizzle the prepared dressing over the salad ingredients.

6. Toss gently to coat everything evenly with the dressing.

7. Serve immediately as a side dish or topped with additional protein for a complete meal.

Nutritional Information (per serving):

- **Calories:** 250 kcal
- **Fat:** 15g
- **Carbohydrates:** 10g
- **Proteins:** 20g

Tuna Salad with Cucumber and Dill

Prep Time: 10 minutes | **Cook Time:** 0 minutes | **Number of Servings:** 4

Ingredients:

- 2 cans (5 oz each) tuna, drained
- 1 cucumber, diced
- 1/4 cup red onion, finely diced
- 1/4 cup fresh dill, chopped
- Juice of 1 lemon
- 2 tablespoons olive oil
- Salt and pepper to taste
- Mixed salad greens for serving

Instructions:

1. In a large bowl, flake the drained tuna with a fork.
2. Add diced cucumber, finely diced red onion, and chopped fresh dill to the bowl.
3. In a small bowl, whisk together lemon juice, olive oil, salt, and pepper to make the dressing.
4. Pour the dressing over the tuna mixture in the large bowl.
5. Toss gently to combine everything evenly.
6. To serve, divide mixed salad greens among plates and top with the tuna salad mixture.

Nutritional Information (per serving):

- **Calories:** 200 kcal
- **Fat:** 10g
- **Carbohydrates:** 5g
- **Proteins:** 25g

Roasted Vegetable and Herb Salad with Chicken

Prep Time: 15 minutes | **Cook Time:** 25 minutes | **Number of Servings:** 4

Ingredients:

- 1-pound chicken breasts, boneless and skinless
- 2 cups cherry tomatoes
- 2 bell peppers, seeded and sliced
- 1 zucchini, sliced
- 1 yellow squash, sliced
- 1 red onion, thinly sliced
- 2 tablespoons olive oil
- 1 teaspoon dried thyme
- 1 teaspoon dried rosemary
- Salt and pepper to taste
- Mixed salad greens for serving
- Fresh herbs (such as parsley or basil) for garnish

Instructions:

1. Preheat oven to 400°F (200°C).

2. Place chicken breasts on a baking sheet. Drizzle with 1 tablespoon olive oil and sprinkle with dried thyme, dried rosemary, salt, and pepper. Rub to coat evenly.

3. In a large bowl, toss cherry tomatoes, bell peppers, zucchini, and yellow squash with remaining 1 tablespoon olive oil. Season with salt and pepper.

4. Spread vegetables evenly on another baking sheet.

5. Place both baking sheets in the preheated oven. Roast chicken for 20-25 minutes or until cooked through (internal temperature of 165°F or 74°C). Roast vegetables for 20 minutes or until tender and slightly caramelized.

6. Remove chicken and vegetables from the oven. Let chicken rest for 5 minutes before slicing.

7. To assemble, divide mixed salad greens among plates.

8. Top with roasted vegetables and sliced chicken breasts.

9. Garnish with fresh herbs.

10. Serve immediately.

Nutritional Information (per serving):

- **Calories:** 350 kcal
- **Fat:** 15g
- **Carbohydrates:** 15g
- **Proteins:** 35g

Mixed Greens Salad with Egg Yolks and Olive Oil Dressing

Prep Time: 10 minutes | **Cook Time:** 0 minutes | **Number of Servings:** 4

Ingredients:

- 8 cups mixed salad greens (such as spinach, arugula, and romaine)
- 4 hard-boiled eggs, yolks separated and reserved
- 1/4 cup olive oil
- 2 tablespoons apple cider vinegar
- Salt and pepper to taste
- Optional: Additional chopped fresh herbs for garnish

Instructions:

1. Prepare the salad greens by washing and drying them thoroughly. Place in a large salad bowl.
2. Separate the hard-boiled egg yolks from the whites. Reserve the yolks.
3. In a small bowl, mash the reserved egg yolks with a fork until smooth.
4. Add olive oil and apple cider vinegar to the mashed egg yolks. Whisk until well combined.
5. Season the dressing with salt and pepper to taste.
6. Pour the dressing over the mixed salad greens in the large bowl.
7. Toss gently to coat the greens evenly with the dressing.
8. To serve, divide the dressed salad among plates.
9. Garnish with additional chopped fresh herbs if desired.

Nutritional Information (per serving):

- **Calories:** 200 kcal
- **Fat:** 15g
- **Carbohydrates:** 5g
- **Proteins:** 10g

<u>Grilled Salmon with Arugula and Pomegranate Seeds</u>

Prep Time: 10 minutes | **Cook Time:** 10 minutes | **Number of Servings:** 4

Ingredients:

- 4 salmon fillets (about 6 oz each), skin-on
- 8 cups arugula
- Seeds from 1 pomegranate

- 1/4 cup chopped walnuts
- Juice of 1 lemon
- 2 tablespoons olive oil
- Salt and pepper to taste

Instructions:

1. Preheat grill to medium-high heat.
2. Season salmon fillets with salt and pepper.
3. Grill salmon fillets, skin-side down, for about 4-5 minutes per side, or until cooked through and flaky. Remove from grill and let rest for a few minutes.
4. In a large bowl, combine arugula, pomegranate seeds, and chopped walnuts.
5. In a small bowl, whisk together lemon juice, olive oil, salt, and pepper to make the dressing.
6. Pour the dressing over the arugula mixture in the large bowl.
7. Toss gently to coat everything evenly with the dressing.
8. To serve, divide the dressed arugula among plates.
9. Place grilled salmon fillets on top of the arugula.
10. Serve immediately.

Nutritional Information (per serving):

- **Calories:** 350 kcal
- **Fat:** 20g
- **Carbohydrates:** 10g
- **Proteins:** 30g

Turkey and Apple Slaw with Carrot-Ginger Dressing

Prep Time: 20 minutes | **Cook Time:** 0 minutes | **Number of Servings:** 4

Ingredients:

- For the Slaw:
    - 1-pound turkey breast, cooked and shredded
    - 2 apples, julienned
    - 2 cups shredded cabbage
    - 1/2 cup shredded carrots
    - 1/4 cup chopped fresh parsley
    - 1/4 cup chopped walnuts (optional)
- For the Dressing:
    - 1/4 cup carrot juice
    - 1 tablespoon fresh ginger, grated
    - 2 tablespoons olive oil
    - Juice of 1 lemon
    - Salt and pepper to taste

Instructions:

1. In a large bowl, combine shredded turkey breast, julienned apples, shredded cabbage, shredded carrots, chopped fresh parsley, and chopped walnuts (if using).

2. In a small bowl, whisk together carrot juice, grated fresh ginger, olive oil, lemon juice, salt, and pepper to make the dressing.

3. Pour the dressing over the turkey and apple slaw mixture in the large bowl.

4. Toss gently to coat everything evenly with the dressing.

5. To serve, divide the slaw among plates.

6. Serve immediately.

Nutritional Information (per serving):

- **Calories:** 300 kcal

- **Fat:** 15g

- **Carbohydrates:** 15g

- **Proteins:** 25g

Zucchini Noodles with Walnut Pesto and Cherry Tomatoes

Prep Time: 15 minutes | **Cook Time:** 10 minutes | **Number of Servings:** 4

Ingredients:

- 4 medium zucchinis, spiralized into noodles
- 1 cup cherry tomatoes, halved
- 1/4 cup chopped walnuts
- Fresh basil leaves for garnish

For the Walnut Pesto:

- 1 cup fresh basil leaves
- 1/2 cup chopped walnuts
- 1/4 cup olive oil
- 2 cloves garlic, minced
- Juice of 1 lemon
- Salt and pepper to taste

Instructions:

1. Make the Walnut Pesto: In a food processor, combine fresh basil leaves, chopped walnuts, olive oil, minced garlic, lemon juice, salt, and pepper. Process until smooth and well combined.

2. In a large skillet, heat a small amount of olive oil over medium heat.

3. Add cherry tomatoes to the skillet and sauté for 2-3 minutes until they begin to soften.

4. Add zucchini noodles to the skillet. Sauté for about 3-4 minutes until zucchini noodles are just tender.

5. Remove skillet from heat and stir in the walnut pesto.

6. To serve, divide the zucchini noodles among plates.

7. Top with chopped walnuts and garnish with fresh basil leaves.

Nutritional Information (per serving):

- **Calories:** 250 kcal
- **Fat:** 20g
- **Carbohydrates:** 10g
- **Proteins:** 8g

Baked Cod with Spinach and Avocado Salsa

Prep Time: 15 minutes | **Cook Time:** 15 minutes | **Number of Servings:** 4

Ingredients:

- 4 cod fillets (about 6 oz each)
- 8 cups fresh spinach leaves
- 2 avocados, diced
- 1/2 cup cherry tomatoes, halved
- 1/4 cup red onion, finely diced
- Juice of 1 lime
- 2 tablespoons olive oil
- Salt and pepper to taste

Instructions:

1. Preheat oven to 400°F (200°C).
2. Place cod fillets on a baking sheet lined with parchment paper.
3. Season cod fillets with salt and pepper.
4. Bake cod fillets in the preheated oven for 12-15 minutes, or until fish is cooked through and flakes easily with a fork.
5. Meanwhile, in a large bowl, combine fresh spinach leaves, diced avocados, halved cherry tomatoes, and finely diced red onion.
6. In a small bowl, whisk together lime juice, olive oil, salt, and pepper to make the dressing.
7. Pour the dressing over the spinach and avocado mixture in the large bowl.
8. Toss gently to coat everything evenly with the dressing.
9. To serve, divide the spinach and avocado salsa among plates.
10. Top each serving with a baked cod fillet.
11. Serve immediately.

Nutritional Information (per serving):

- **Calories:** 300 kcal
- **Fat:** 15g
- **Carbohydrates:** 10g
- **Proteins:** 30g

Dinner Recipes

Herb-Roasted Chicken with Brussels Sprouts

- **Prep Time:** 15 minutes | **Cook Time:** 40 minutes | **Servings:** 4

Ingredients:

- 4 bone-in, skin-on chicken thighs
- 1-pound Brussels sprouts, halved
- 2 tablespoons olive oil
- 2 cloves garlic, minced
- 1 teaspoon dried thyme
- 1 teaspoon dried rosemary
- 1 teaspoon dried oregano
- Salt and pepper, to taste
- Fresh parsley, chopped (for garnish)

Instructions:

1. Preheat your oven to 400°F (200°C).
2. Prepare the chicken thighs by patting them dry with paper towels. Season generously with salt and pepper.
3. In a large bowl, combine the Brussels sprouts, olive oil, minced garlic, dried thyme, dried rosemary, and dried oregano. Toss until the Brussels sprouts are evenly coated.
4. Arrange the seasoned Brussels sprouts on a baking sheet in an even layer.
5. Place the seasoned chicken thighs on top of the Brussels sprouts on the baking sheet.
6. Roast in the preheated oven for 35-40 minutes, or until the chicken reaches an internal temperature of 165°F (74°C) and the Brussels sprouts are tender and caramelized.
7. Remove from the oven and let rest for 5 minutes before serving.
8. Garnish with chopped fresh parsley before serving.

Nutritional Information (per serving):

- **Calories:** 380 kcal
- **Fat:** 21 g
- **Carbohydrates:** 12 g
- **Protein:** 34 g

Baked Salmon with Asparagus and Lemon Dill Sauce

- **Prep Time:** 15 minutes | **Cook Time:** 15 minutes | **Servings:** 4

Ingredients:

- 4 salmon fillets (about 6 oz each), skin-on
- 1-pound asparagus spears, tough ends trimmed
- 2 tablespoons olive oil
- Salt and pepper, to taste

- For the Lemon Dill Sauce:
  - 1/2 cup coconut milk
  - Zest and juice of 1 lemon
  - 1 tablespoon fresh dill, chopped
  - Salt and pepper, to taste

Instructions:

1. Preheat your oven to 400°F (200°C).

2. Place the asparagus spears on a baking sheet. Drizzle with 1 tablespoon of olive oil, season with salt and pepper, and toss to coat evenly.

3. Season the salmon fillets with salt and pepper on both sides. Place the salmon fillets skin-side down on the baking sheet with the asparagus.

4. Bake in the preheated oven for 12-15 minutes, or until the salmon is cooked through and flakes easily with a fork, and the asparagus is tender.

5. In a small saucepan, combine the coconut milk, lemon zest, lemon juice, and chopped dill. Heat gently over low heat, stirring occasionally, until warmed through. Season with salt and pepper to taste.

6. Serve the baked salmon and asparagus hot, drizzled with the Lemon Dill Sauce.

Nutritional Information (per serving):

- **Calories:** 380 kcal
- **Fat:** 24 g
- **Carbohydrates:** 7 g
- **Protein:** 34 g

Beef and Vegetable Stew with Sweet Potatoes

- **Prep Time:** 20 minutes | **Cook Time:** 2 hours | **Servings:** 6

Ingredients:

- 1.5 pounds beef stew meat, cubed
- 2 tablespoons olive oil
- 1 onion, diced
- 2 cloves garlic, minced
- 3 carrots, peeled and sliced
- 2 celery stalks, sliced
- 2 medium sweet potatoes, peeled and cubed
- 4 cups beef broth
- 1 teaspoon dried thyme
- 1 teaspoon dried rosemary
- Salt and pepper, to taste
- Fresh parsley, chopped (for garnish)

Instructions:

1. Heat 1 tablespoon of olive oil in a large pot or Dutch oven over medium-high heat. Add the cubed beef stew meat and cook until browned on all sides. Take out the beef from the pot and set aside.

2. Add the remaining tablespoon of olive oil to the pot. Add the diced onion and minced garlic, sautéing until softened and fragrant.

3. Stir in the sliced carrots, sliced celery, and cubed sweet potatoes. Cook for about 5 minutes, stirring occasionally.

4. Return the browned beef to the pot. Pour in the beef broth, and add the dried thyme and dried rosemary. Season with salt and pepper to taste.

5. Bring the stew to a boil, then reduce the heat to low. Cover and simmer for about 1.5 to 2 hours, or until the beef is tender and the sweet potatoes are cooked through.

6. Adjust seasoning if needed. Serve hot, garnished with chopped fresh parsley.

Nutritional Information (per serving):

- **Calories:** 380 kcal
- **Fat:** 14 g
- **Carbohydrates:** 28 g
- **Protein:** 32 g

Pork Tenderloin with Apple Compote and Roasted Carrots

- **Prep Time:** 15 minutes | **Cook Time:** 30 minutes | **Servings:** 4

Ingredients:

- 1-pound pork tenderloin
- 2 tablespoons olive oil, divided
- Salt and pepper, to taste
- For the Apple Compote:
    - 2 apples, peeled, cored, and chopped
- For the Roasted Carrots:
    - 1-pound carrots, peeled and cut into sticks

- 1 tablespoon ghee or coconut oil
- 1 tablespoon honey (optional, omit for strict AIP)
- 1/2 teaspoon ground cinnamon

- 1 tablespoon olive oil
- Salt and pepper, to taste

Instructions:

1. Preheat your oven to 400°F (200°C).

2. Prepare the pork tenderloin by patting it dry with paper towels. Season with salt and pepper on all sides.

3. Heat 1 tablespoon of olive oil in an oven-safe skillet over medium-high heat. Sear the pork tenderloin on all sides until browned, about 2-3 minutes per side.

4. Transfer the skillet to the preheated oven. Roast the pork tenderloin for 15-20 minutes, or until it reaches an internal temperature of 145°F (63°C). Remove from the oven and let rest for 5 minutes before slicing.

5. In a saucepan, heat the ghee or coconut oil over medium heat. Add the chopped apples, honey (if using), and ground cinnamon. Cook until the apples are softened and caramelized, about 8-10 minutes. Mash lightly with a fork or potato masher.

6. Toss the carrot sticks with 1 tablespoon of olive oil, salt, and pepper on a baking sheet. Roast in the preheated oven for 20-25 minutes, or until tender and lightly caramelized.

7. Slice the pork tenderloin into medallions. Serve hot, topped with the Apple Compote and alongside the Roasted Carrots.

Nutritional Information (per serving):

- **Calories:** 360 kcal
- **Fat:** 16 g
- **Carbohydrates:** 22 g
- **Protein:** 32 g

Lemon-Garlic Shrimp with Zucchini Noodles

- **Prep Time:** 15 minutes | **Cook Time:** 10 minutes | **Servings:** 4

Ingredients:

- 1-pound large shrimp, peeled and deveined
- 4 medium zucchini, spiralized into noodles
- 3 tablespoons olive oil, divided
- 4 cloves garlic, minced
- Zest and juice of 1 lemon
- 1/2 teaspoon red pepper flakes (optional)
- Salt and pepper, to taste
- Fresh parsley, chopped (for garnish)

Instructions:

1. Heat 2 tablespoons of olive oil in a large skillet over medium-high heat.

2. Add the minced garlic and red pepper flakes (if using). Sauté for about 1 minute until fragrant.

3. Add the shrimp to the skillet in a single layer. Cook for 2-3 minutes per side, or until shrimp are pink and opaque. Take out the shrimp from the skillet and set aside.

4. In the same skillet, add the remaining tablespoon of olive oil. Add the zucchini noodles and lemon zest. Sauté for 2-3 minutes, tossing gently, until the noodles are just tender but still crisp.

5. Return the cooked shrimp to the skillet with the zucchini noodles. Add the lemon juice and toss everything together until well combined and heated through. Season with salt and pepper to taste.

6. Serve hot, garnished with chopped fresh parsley.

Nutritional Information (per serving):

- **Calories:** 280 kcal
- **Fat:** 12 g
- **Carbohydrates:** 10 g
- **Protein:** 32 g

Lamb Chops with Mint and Roasted Root Vegetables

- **Prep Time:** 15 minutes | **Cook Time:** 30 minutes | **Servings:** 4

Ingredients:

- 8 lamb loin chops
- 2 tablespoons olive oil, divided
- Salt and pepper, to taste
- For the Mint Sauce:

  - 1/2 cup fresh mint leaves, chopped
  - 2 tablespoons olive oil
  - 1 tablespoon lemon juice
  - Salt and pepper, to taste

- For the Roasted Root Vegetables:

  - 1-pound mixed root vegetables (such as carrots, parsnips, and turnips), peeled and cut into chunks
  - 1 tablespoon olive oil
  - 1 teaspoon dried thyme
  - 1 teaspoon dried rosemary
  - Salt and pepper, to taste

Instructions:

1. Preheat your oven to 400°F (200°C).
2. Prepare the lamb chops by patting them dry with paper towels. Season with salt and pepper on both sides.
3. Heat 1 tablespoon of olive oil in a large oven-safe skillet over medium-high heat. Sear the lamb chops for 3-4 minutes per side until browned. Remove from the skillet and set aside.
4. In a small bowl, combine the chopped mint leaves, 2 tablespoons of olive oil, lemon juice, salt, and pepper. Set aside.
5. In a large bowl, toss the peeled and cut root vegetables with 1 tablespoon of olive oil, dried thyme, dried rosemary, salt, and pepper until evenly coated. Spread them out on a baking sheet in a single layer.
6. Roast the root vegetables in the preheated oven for 20-25 minutes, or until they are tender and lightly caramelized.
7. Meanwhile, return the seared lamb chops to the skillet (if using an oven-safe skillet) or transfer them to a baking dish. Place them in the oven and roast for 10-12 minutes for medium-rare, or longer according to your preference.
8. Serve the roasted lamb chops hot, topped with the Mint Sauce, alongside the Roasted Root Vegetables.

Nutritional Information (per serving):

- **Calories:** 420 kcal
- **Fat:** 24 g
- **Carbohydrates:** 12 g
- **Protein:** 38 g

Grilled Steak with Chimichurri Sauce and Cauliflower Rice

- **Prep Time:** 20 minutes | **Cook Time:** 15 minutes | **Servings:** 4

Ingredients:

- 4 beef sirloin or ribeye steaks, about 6 oz each
- 1 large head cauliflower, grated into rice-like texture
  - 1 cup fresh parsley leaves, chopped
  - 1/2 cup fresh cilantro leaves, chopped
- 2 tablespoons olive oil, divided
- Salt and pepper, to taste
- For the Chimichurri Sauce:
  - 2 cloves garlic, minced
  - 1/4 cup red wine vinegar
  - 1/2 cup olive oil
  - Salt and pepper, to taste

Instructions:

1. Preheat your grill to medium-high heat.

2. Prepare the steaks by patting them dry with paper towels. Brush each steak with 1 tablespoon of olive oil and season with salt and pepper on both sides.

3. Grill the steaks for about 4-5 minutes per side, or until they reach your desired level of doneness (145°F or 63°C for medium-rare). Remove from the grill and let rest for 5 minutes before slicing.

4. In a bowl, combine the chopped parsley, chopped cilantro, minced garlic, red wine vinegar, and olive oil. Season with salt and pepper to taste. Set aside.

5. Grate the head of cauliflower using a box grater or a food processor until it resembles rice grains.

6. Heat 1 tablespoon of olive oil in a large skillet over medium heat. Add the grated cauliflower rice and sauté for about 5-7 minutes, stirring frequently, until it is tender but still slightly crisp. Season with salt and pepper to taste.

7. Serve the grilled steaks hot, topped with Chimichurri Sauce, alongside the Cauliflower Rice.

Nutritional Information (per serving):

- **Calories:** 420 kcal
- **Fat:** 26 g
- **Carbohydrates:** 10 g
- **Protein:** 38 g

<u>Coconut Chicken Curry with Cauliflower Rice</u>

- **Prep Time:** 20 minutes | **Cook Time:** 30 minutes | **Servings:** 4

Ingredients:

- 1.5 pounds boneless, skinless chicken breasts, cut into bite-sized pieces
- 2 tablespoons coconut oil, divided
- 1 onion, finely chopped
- 3 cloves garlic, minced
- 1 tablespoon ginger, minced
- 1 red bell pepper, diced
- 1 tablespoon curry powder
- 1 teaspoon ground turmeric
- 1/2 teaspoon ground cumin
- 1/2 teaspoon ground coriander

- 1/4 teaspoon cayenne pepper (optional, adjust to taste)
- 1 can (14 oz) coconut milk
- 1 cup chicken broth
- 2 tablespoons tomato paste
- Salt and pepper, to taste
- Fresh cilantro, chopped (for garnish)
- ***For the Cauliflower Rice:***
  - 1 large head cauliflower, grated into rice-like texture
  - 1 tablespoon coconut oil
  - Salt and pepper, to taste

Instructions:

1. Heat 1 tablespoon of coconut oil in a large skillet or Dutch oven over medium-high heat. Add the chicken pieces and cook until browned on all sides. Take out the chicken from the skillet and set aside.
2. Add the remaining tablespoon of coconut oil to the skillet. Add the chopped onion, minced garlic, and minced ginger. Sauté for about 3-4 minutes, until the onions are fragrant.
3. Stir in the diced red bell pepper, curry powder, ground turmeric, ground cumin, ground coriander, and cayenne pepper (if using). Cook for another 2 minutes, stirring constantly, until the spices are fragrant.
4. Pour in the coconut milk, chicken broth, and tomato paste. Stir adequately to combine, scraping up any browned bits from the bottom of the skillet.
5. Return the browned chicken pieces to the skillet. Bring the mixture to a boil, then reduce the heat to low and let it simmer for 15-20 minutes, or until the chicken is cooked through and the sauce has thickened slightly. Season with salt and pepper to taste.
6. Grate the head of cauliflower using a box grater until it resembles rice grains.
7. Heat 1 tablespoon of coconut oil in a large skillet over medium heat. Add the grated cauliflower rice and sauté for about 5-7 minutes, stirring frequently, until it is tender but still slightly crisp. Season with salt and pepper to taste.
8. Serve the Coconut Chicken Curry hot, garnished with chopped fresh cilantro, alongside the Cauliflower Rice.

Nutritional Information (per serving):

- **Calories:** 420 kcal
- **Protein:** 40 g
- **Fat:** 25 g
- **Carbohydrates:** 10 g

AIP Meatloaf with Mashed Parsnips

- **Prep Time:** 20 minutes | **Cook Time:** 1 hour | **Servings:** 6

Ingredients:

- ***For the Meatloaf:***

  - 1-pound ground beef (preferably grass-fed)
  - 1-pound ground pork
  - 1 onion, finely chopped
  - 2 cloves garlic, minced
  - 1/2 cup chopped fresh parsley
  - 1/2 cup chopped fresh cilantro
  - 1 tablespoon dried oregano
  - 1 tablespoon dried thyme
  - 2 tablespoons coconut aminos
  - 2 tablespoons olive oil
  - Salt and pepper, to taste

- ***For the Mashed Parsnips:***

  - 2 pounds parsnips, peeled and cut into chunks
  - 1/4 cup coconut milk (full-fat)
  - 2 tablespoons ghee (omit for strict AIP)
  - Salt, to taste

Instructions:

1. Preheat your oven to 375°F (190°C).

2. In a large bowl, combine the ground beef, ground pork, chopped onion, minced garlic, chopped parsley, chopped cilantro, dried oregano, dried thyme, coconut aminos, olive oil, salt, and pepper. Mix until well combined.

3. Transfer the meat mixture into a loaf pan, pressing it down evenly.

4. Bake the meatloaf in the preheated oven for 50-60 minutes, or until cooked through and the internal temperature reaches 160°F (71°C). Remove from the oven and let it rest for 10 minutes before slicing.

5. While the meatloaf is baking, place the peeled and chopped parsnips in a large pot. Cover with water and bring to a boil. Cook for 15-20 minutes, or until the parsnips are tender when pierced with a fork.

6. Drain the cooked parsnips and return them to the pot.

7. Mash the parsnips using a potato masher or fork until smooth.

8. Add the coconut milk and ghee (if using) to the mashed parsnips. Continue mashing until well combined and creamy. Season with salt to taste.

9. Serve slices of the Meatloaf hot, accompanied by a generous serving of Mashed Parsnips.

Nutritional Information (per serving):

- **Calories:** 480 kcal
- **Fat:** 28 g
- **Carbohydrates:** 20 g
- **Protein:** 35 g

<u>Ginger-Turmeric Chicken Thighs with Broccoli</u>

- **Prep Time:** 15 minutes | **Cook Time:** 25 minutes | **Servings:** 4

Ingredients:

- 4 bone-in, skin-on chicken thighs
- 1 tablespoon coconut oil, melted
- 1 tablespoon fresh ginger, grated
- 1 tablespoon ground turmeric
- 1 teaspoon ground cumin
- 1/2 teaspoon ground coriander
- 1/4 teaspoon cayenne pepper (optional, adjust to taste)
- Salt and pepper, to taste
- 1-pound broccoli florets
- 2 tablespoons olive oil
- Lemon wedges (for serving)

Instructions:

1. Preheat your oven to 400°F (200°C).
2. Place the chicken thighs on a baking sheet lined with parchment paper.
3. In a small bowl, combine the melted coconut oil, grated ginger, ground turmeric, ground cumin, ground coriander, cayenne pepper (if using), salt, and pepper. Mix adequately.
4. Brush the ginger-turmeric mixture evenly over the chicken thighs, coating both sides.
5. Roast the chicken thighs in the preheated oven for 20-25 minutes, or until the internal temperature reaches 165°F (74°C) and the skin is crispy.
6. While the chicken thighs are roasting, toss the broccoli florets with olive oil, salt, and pepper on another baking sheet.
7. Arrange the broccoli in a single layer and roast in the oven alongside the chicken thighs for about 15-20 minutes, or until tender and lightly browned.
8. Serve the Ginger-Turmeric Chicken Thighs hot, accompanied by roasted broccoli and lemon wedges for squeezing.

Nutritional Information (per serving):

- **Calories:** 380 kcal
- **Fat:** 24 g
- **Carbohydrates:** 10 g
- **Protein:** 32 g

Baked Cod with Almond Crust and Green Beans

- **Prep Time:** 15 minutes | **Cook Time:** 20 minutes | **Servings:** 4

Ingredients:

- 4 cod fillets (about 6 oz each), skinless
- 1 cup almond flour
- 1/2 cup sliced almonds
- 1 teaspoon garlic powder
- 1 teaspoon onion powder
- 1/2 teaspoon paprika
- Salt and pepper, to taste
- 2 eggs, beaten
- 1-pound green beans, trimmed
- Olive oil cooking spray

Instructions:

1. Preheat your oven to 400°F (200°C). Line a baking sheet with parchment paper.
2. In a shallow bowl, combine the almond flour, sliced almonds, garlic powder, onion powder, paprika, salt, and pepper.
3. Dip each cod fillet into the beaten eggs, then dredge in the almond mixture, pressing gently to adhere. Place the coated fillets on the prepared baking sheet.
4. Bake the cod in the preheated oven for 15-20 minutes, or until the fish is opaque and flakes easily with a fork.
5. While the cod is baking, steam or boil the green beans until tender-crisp, about 5-7 minutes. Drain and set aside.
6. Serve the Baked Cod hot, accompanied by steamed green beans.

Nutritional Information (per serving):

- **Calories:** 380 kcal
- **Fat:** 22 g
- **Carbohydrates:** 12 g
- **Protein:** 34 g

Stuffed Bell Peppers with Ground Beef and Vegetables

- **Prep Time:** 20 minutes | **Cook Time:** 40 minutes | **Servings:** 4

Ingredients:

- 4 large bell peppers (any color), tops removed and seeds removed
- 1-pound ground beef (preferably grass-fed)
- 1 onion, finely chopped
- 2 cloves garlic, minced
- 1 carrot, finely diced
- 1 celery stalk, finely diced
- 1 zucchini, finely diced
- 1/2 cup tomato sauce
- 1 teaspoon dried oregano
- 1 teaspoon dried basil
- Salt and pepper, to taste
- Olive oil, for cooking

Instructions:

1. Preheat your oven to 375°F (190°C).
2. Place the bell peppers upright in a baking dish. If necessary, slice a small piece off the bottom to help them stand upright without tipping over. Set aside.
3. In a large skillet, heat a drizzle of olive oil over medium-high heat. Add the ground beef and cook until browned, breaking it up with a spoon as it cooks.
4. Add the chopped onion, minced garlic, diced carrot, diced celery, and diced zucchini to the skillet with the ground beef. Cook for about 5-7 minutes, or until the vegetables are softened.
5. Stir in the tomato sauce, dried oregano, dried basil, salt, and pepper. Cook for another 2-3 minutes, stirring occasionally, until heated through.
6. Stuff each bell pepper with the ground beef and vegetable mixture, pressing gently to pack the filling.
7. Cover the baking dish with foil and bake in the preheated oven for 30 minutes.
8. Uncover the baking dish and bake for an additional 10 minutes, or until the bell peppers are tender.
9. Serve the Stuffed Bell Peppers hot, optionally garnished with fresh herbs.

Nutritional Information (per serving):

- **Calories:** 380 kcal
- **Fat:** 20 g
- **Carbohydrates:** 15 g
- **Protein:** 32 g

Snacks Recipes

Apple Slices with Almond Butter

Prep Time: 10 minutes | **Cook Time:** N/A | **Number of Servings:** 2

Ingredients:

- 1 medium apple, cored and sliced
- 4 tablespoons almond butter
- 1 tablespoon unsweetened shredded coconut
- 1 tablespoon chopped almonds

Instructions:

1. Core the apple and slice it into thin wedges.
2. Spread almond butter evenly on each apple slice.
3. Sprinkle shredded coconut and chopped almonds over the almond butter.
4. Arrange the apple slices on a serving plate and enjoy immediately.

Nutritional Information:

- **Calories:** 180 kcal per serving
- **Fat:** 10g
- **Carbs:** 16g
- **Proteins:** 5g

Carrot and Celery Sticks with AIP Ranch Dip

Prep Time: 15 minutes | **Cook Time:** N/A | **Number of Servings:** 4

Ingredients:

- 2 large carrots, peeled and cut into sticks
- 4 celery stalks, cut into sticks
- For the AIP Ranch Dip:
    - 1/2 cup coconut milk (full fat)
    - 1 tablespoon fresh lemon juice
    - 1/2 teaspoon onion powder
    - 1/2 teaspoon garlic powder
    - 1/2 teaspoon dried dill
    - Salt, to taste
    - Freshly ground black pepper, to taste (optional)

Instructions:

1. Peel the carrots and cut them into sticks.
2. Wash the celery stalks and cut them into sticks.
3. In a small bowl, whisk together coconut milk, lemon juice, onion powder, garlic powder, and dried dill until well combined.
4. Season with salt and optionally, pepper, to taste.
5. Arrange the carrot and celery sticks on a serving plate.
6. Serve with the AIP Ranch Dip on the side for dipping.

Nutritional Information:

- **Calories:** 120 kcal per serving
- **Fat:** 8g
- **Carbs:** 10g
- **Proteins:** 2g

Homemade AIP Granola Bars with Pumpkin Seeds

Prep Time: 15 minutes | **Cook Time:** 20 minutes | **Number of Servings:** 8 bars

Ingredients:

- 1 cup shredded unsweetened coconut
- 1 cup pumpkin seeds
- 1/2 cup sunflower seeds
- 1/2 cup dried cranberries (unsweetened)
- 1/4 cup coconut oil, melted
- 1/4 cup honey (or maple syrup for strict AIP)
- 1 teaspoon vanilla extract
- Pinch of salt

Instructions:

1. Preheat your oven to 350°F (175°C). Line a baking dish with parchment paper.
2. In a large bowl, combine shredded coconut, pumpkin seeds, sunflower seeds, and dried cranberries.
3. In a small bowl, whisk together melted coconut oil, honey (or maple syrup), vanilla extract, and a pinch of salt.
4. Pour the wet ingredients over the dry ingredients in the large bowl. Mix until everything is evenly coated.
5. Transfer the mixture into the lined baking dish. Press it down firmly and evenly with a spatula.
6. Bake in the preheated oven for about 20 minutes, or until the edges are golden brown.
7. Remove from the oven and let it cool completely in the baking dish.
8. Once cooled, lift the granola slab using the parchment paper and cut it into 8 bars.

Nutritional Information:

- **Calories:** 250 kcal per bar
- **Fat:** 18g
- **Carbs:** 20g
- **Proteins:** 5g

Baked Kale Chips with Sea Salt

Prep Time: 10 minutes | **Cook Time:** 15 minutes | **Number of Servings:** 4

Ingredients:

- 1 bunch kale
- 1 tablespoon olive oil
- Sea salt, to taste

Instructions:

1. Preheat your oven to 350°F (175°C). Line a baking sheet with parchment paper.
2. Wash the kale leaves thoroughly and pat them dry with a paper towel. Take out the tough stems and tear the leaves into bite-sized pieces.
3. In a large bowl, toss the kale pieces with olive oil until evenly coated. Massage the oil into the kale leaves to ensure they are well coated.
4. Spread the kale pieces in a single layer on the prepared baking sheet.
5. Sprinkle sea salt evenly over the kale chips.
6. Bake in the preheated oven for about 12-15 minutes, or until the edges are crispy and slightly browned. Watch carefully to prevent burning.
7. Remove from the oven and let the kale chips cool on the baking sheet for a few minutes.
8. Transfer to a serving bowl and serve immediately.

Nutritional Information:

- **Calories:** 50 kcal per serving
- **Fat:** 3g
- **Carbs:** 5g
- **Proteins:** 2g

Coconut Macaroons with Dark Chocolate Drizzle

Prep Time: 15 minutes | **Cook Time:** 20 minutes | **Number of Servings:** 12 macaroons

Ingredients:

- 2 cups unsweetened shredded coconut
- 1/2 cup coconut butter, melted
- 1/4 cup honey (or maple syrup for strict AIP)
- 1 teaspoon vanilla extract
- Pinch of salt
- 1/2 cup dark chocolate chips (at least 70% cocoa), melted

Instructions:

1. Preheat your oven to 325°F (160°C). Line a baking sheet with parchment paper.
2. In a large bowl, combine shredded coconut, melted coconut butter, honey (or maple syrup), vanilla extract, and a pinch of salt. Mix until well combined.
3. Take about 2 tablespoons of the mixture and shape it into a ball using your hands. Place it on the prepared baking sheet. Repeat with the remaining mixture, spacing the macaroons evenly apart.
4. Bake in the preheated oven for about 18-20 minutes, or until the macaroons are lightly golden brown around the edges.
5. Remove from the oven and let the macaroons cool completely on the baking sheet.
6. Melt the dark chocolate chips in a microwave-safe bowl in 30-second intervals, stirring in between, until smooth.
7. Drizzle melted dark chocolate over the cooled macaroons using a spoon or piping bag.
8. Allow the chocolate to set at room temperature, then transfer the macaroons to a serving plate.

Nutritional Information:

- **Calories:** 180 kcal per macaroon
- **Fat:** 14g
- **Carbs:** 12g
- **Proteins:** 2g

Deviled Eggs with Avocado and Paprika

Prep Time: 20 minutes | **Cook Time:** 10 minutes | **Number of Servings:** 6 eggs (12 halves)

Ingredients:

- 6 large eggs
- 1 ripe avocado
- 2 tablespoons mayonnaise (check for AIP compliance or use homemade)
- 1 tablespoon fresh lemon juice
- 1/2 teaspoon onion powder
- 1/2 teaspoon garlic powder
- Salt and pepper, to taste
- Paprika, for garnish

Instructions:

1. Place the eggs in a single layer in a saucepan and cover with water. Bring to a boil over medium-high heat.
2. Once boiling, remove from heat, cover, and let the eggs sit in hot water for 10 minutes.
3. Drain the hot water and rinse the eggs under cold water. Peel the eggs and cut them in half lengthwise. Take out the yolks and set aside.
4. Scoop out the flesh of the avocado and place it in a bowl. Mash the avocado with a fork until smooth.
5. To the mashed avocado, add the reserved egg yolks, mayonnaise, lemon juice, onion powder, garlic powder, salt, and pepper. Mix until well combined and creamy.
6. Spoon or pipe the avocado mixture into the hollowed-out egg whites, dividing evenly among the egg halves.
7. Sprinkle paprika over the filled deviled eggs for garnish.

Nutritional Information:

- **Calories:** 100 kcal per 2 halves
- **Fat:** 7g
- **Carbs:** 3g
- **Proteins:** 5g

Mixed Berry Fruit Leather

Prep Time: 15 minutes | **Cook Time:** 4-6 hours drying time | **Number of Servings:** 8 servings

Ingredients:

- 4 cups mixed berries (such as strawberries, blueberries, raspberries)
- 1 tablespoon honey (optional, adjust to taste)
- 1 tablespoon lemon juice

Instructions:

1. Preheat your oven to the lowest temperature setting, typically around 140-170°F (60-75°C). Line a baking sheet with parchment paper.
2. Wash the mixed berries and pat them dry with a paper towel. Remove any stems.
3. In a blender or food processor, puree the berries until smooth.
4. Taste the berry puree. If desired, add honey to sweeten, adjusting to taste. Add lemon juice for a bit of tartness and to help preserve the color.
5. Pour the berry puree onto the prepared baking sheet. Use a spatula to spread it evenly into a thin layer, about 1/8 inch thick.
6. Place the baking sheet in the preheated oven and prop the oven door open slightly to allow moisture to escape. This helps in drying the fruit leather.
7. Dry for 4-6 hours, or until the fruit leather is dry to the touch and no longer sticky.
8. Remove from the oven and let the fruit leather cool completely on the baking sheet.
9. Once cooled, peel the fruit leather off the parchment paper and cut it into strips or squares.
10. Roll the fruit leather strips with parchment paper and store in an airtight container at room temperature for up to 2 weeks.

Nutritional Information:

- **Calories:** 50 kcal per serving
- **Fat:** 0.5g
- **Carbs:** 12g
- **Proteins:** 1g

Plantain Chips with Guacamole

Prep Time: 15 minutes | **Cook Time:** 20 minutes | **Number of Servings:** 4 servings

Ingredients:

- 2 ripe plantains
- 2 tablespoons olive oil
- Sea salt, to taste

For the Guacamole:

- 2 ripe avocados
- 1 tablespoon lime juice
- 1/4 cup diced tomatoes
- 1/4 cup diced red onion
- 1 tablespoon chopped fresh cilantro
- Salt and pepper, to taste

Instructions:

1. Preheat your oven to 400°F (200°C). Line a baking sheet with parchment paper.
2. Peel the plantains and slice them thinly using a mandoline slicer or a sharp knife.
3. In a bowl, toss the plantain slices with olive oil until evenly coated.
4. Arrange the plantain slices in a single layer on the prepared baking sheet. Sprinkle with sea salt.
5. Bake for about 15-20 minutes, flipping halfway through, until the plantain chips are golden brown and crispy. Watch them closely to prevent burning.
6. While the plantain chips are baking, prepare the guacamole.
7. In a bowl, mash the avocados with a fork until smooth.
8. Stir in lime juice, diced tomatoes, diced red onion, chopped cilantro, salt, and pepper. Mix until well combined.
9. Arrange the plantain chips on a serving platter.
10. Serve with the guacamole on the side for dipping.

Nutritional Information:

- **Calories:** 250 kcal per serving
- **Fat:** 15g
- **Carbs:** 30g
- **Proteins:** 3g

AIP Beef Jerky with Herbs

Prep Time: 20 minutes | **Cook Time:** 4-6 hours drying time | **Number of Servings:** 6 servings

Ingredients:

- 1-pound lean beef (such as top round or flank steak), thinly sliced against the grain
- 2 tablespoons coconut aminos
- 1 tablespoon apple cider vinegar
- 1 tablespoon olive oil
- 1 teaspoon onion powder
- 1 teaspoon garlic powder
- 1/2 teaspoon dried thyme
- 1/2 teaspoon dried oregano
- Salt and pepper, to taste (optional)

Instructions:

1. Trim any visible fat from the beef and slice it thinly against the grain. This helps in making the jerky easier to chew.
2. In a bowl, combine coconut aminos, apple cider vinegar, olive oil, onion powder, garlic powder, dried thyme, dried oregano, salt, and pepper (if using).
3. Add the sliced beef to the marinade, ensuring all pieces are coated evenly. Cover and refrigerate for at least 1 hour, or overnight for best results.
4. Preheat your oven to the lowest temperature setting, typically around 170°F (75°C), or use a food dehydrator according to manufacturer's instructions.
5. Line a baking sheet with parchment paper or use dehydrator trays.
6. Arrange the marinated beef slices in a single layer on the prepared baking sheet or dehydrator trays, ensuring they do not overlap.
7. For oven method: Place the baking sheet in the preheated oven and prop the oven door open slightly to allow moisture to escape. Dry for 4-6 hours, flipping the beef slices halfway through, until the jerky is dry and chewy.
8. For dehydrator method: Follow the manufacturer's instructions for drying meat until the jerky is dry and chewy.
9. Once dried, take out the beef jerky from the oven or dehydrator and let it cool completely.
10. Store the beef jerky in an airtight container at room temperature for up to 2 weeks.

Nutritional Information:

- **Calories:** 150 kcal per serving (about 1 ounce)
- **Fat:** 7g
- **Carbs:** 2g
- **Proteins:** 20g

Chia Seed Pudding with Coconut Milk and Honey

Prep Time: 5 minutes | **Cook Time:** 0 minutes (plus chilling time) | **Number of Servings:** 2 servings

Ingredients:

- 1/4 cup chia seeds

- 1 cup coconut milk (full-fat, canned)

- 1 tablespoon honey (or maple syrup for strict AIP)

- 1/2 teaspoon vanilla extract

- Fresh berries or shredded coconut, for topping (optional)

Instructions:

1. In a bowl or jar, combine chia seeds, coconut milk, honey (or maple syrup), and vanilla extract. Stir adequately to combine all ingredients thoroughly.
2. Cover the bowl or jar and refrigerate for at least 2 hours, or preferably overnight, to allow the chia seeds to absorb the liquid and thicken into pudding consistency.
3. After chilling, stir the chia seed pudding to redistribute the seeds evenly. If desired, add a little more coconut milk to adjust the consistency.
4. Serve the chia seed pudding in individual bowls or jars.
5. Top with fresh berries or shredded coconut, if using, for added flavor and texture.

Nutritional Information:

- **Calories:** 250 kcal per serving

- **Fat:** 20g

- **Carbs:** 15g

- **Proteins:** 5g

Sliced Cucumbers with Smoked Salmon and Dill

Prep Time: 10 minutes | **Cook Time:** 0 minutes | **Number of Servings:** 2 servings

Ingredients:

- 1 large cucumber, thinly sliced
- 4 ounces smoked salmon, sliced
- Fresh dill sprigs, for garnish

Instructions:

1. Wash the cucumber thoroughly and slice it thinly using a sharp knife or a mandoline slicer.
2. Arrange the cucumber slices on a serving platter or individual plates.
3. Place the slices of smoked salmon on top of the cucumber slices, distributing evenly.
4. Garnish with fresh dill sprigs for added flavor and presentation.
5. Serve immediately as a refreshing and nutritious snack or appetizer.

Nutritional Information:

- **Calories:** 180 kcal per serving
- **Fat:** 8g
- **Carbs:** 5g
- **Proteins:** 20g

<u>Trail Mix with Nuts and Dried Fruit</u>

Prep Time: 10 minutes | **Cook Time:** 0 minutes | **Number of Servings:** 6 servings

Ingredients:

- 1 cup mixed nuts (such as almonds, walnuts, cashews)
- 1/2 cup dried fruit (such as cranberries, raisins, apricots)
- 1/4 cup coconut flakes
- 1/4 cup pumpkin seeds (pepitas)
- 1/4 cup sunflower seeds
- 1/4 teaspoon sea salt

Instructions:

1. If using whole nuts, roughly chop them into smaller pieces. Ensure the dried fruit is diced if large pieces.
2. In a large bowl, combine the mixed nuts, dried fruit, coconut flakes, pumpkin seeds, sunflower seeds, and sea salt. Mix adequately to evenly distribute ingredients.
3. Transfer the trail mix to an airtight container or individual snack bags for easy access.

Nutritional Information:

- **Calories:** 250 kcal per serving
- **Fat:** 15g
- **Carbs:** 25g
- **Proteins:** 7g

Chapter 6: Personalization Phase Recipes

Breakfast Recipes

Sweet Potato and Spinach Breakfast Hash

Prep Time: 15 minutes | **Cook Time:** 25 minutes | **Servings:** 4

Ingredients:

- 2 medium sweet potatoes, peeled and diced
- 1 medium onion, diced
- 2 cups fresh spinach, chopped
- 1 red bell pepper, diced
- 2 tablespoons olive oil
- 1 teaspoon dried thyme
- 1 teaspoon dried rosemary
- 1 teaspoon sea salt
- 1/2 teaspoon ground black pepper
- 1/2 pound cooked chicken breast, diced

Instructions:

1. Preheat your oven to 400 degrees Fahrenheit (200 degrees Celsius).

2. In a large bowl, toss the peeled and diced sweet potatoes with one tablespoon of olive oil, 1/2 teaspoon of dried thyme, 1/2 teaspoon of dried rosemary, 1/2 teaspoon of sea salt, and 1/4 teaspoon of ground black pepper.

3. Spread the seasoned sweet potatoes evenly on a baking sheet. Roast in the preheated oven for about 20 minutes or until they are tender and slightly caramelized.

4. While the sweet potatoes are roasting, heat the remaining one tablespoon of olive oil in a large skillet over medium heat. Add the diced onion and diced red bell pepper to the skillet. Sauté for about 5 minutes, or until the onion becomes translucent.

5. Stir in the chopped fresh spinach and cook until it is wilted, about 2-3 minutes.

6. Add the roasted sweet potatoes and the diced cooked chicken breast to the skillet with the vegetables. Stir in the remaining 1/2 teaspoon of dried thyme, 1/2 teaspoon of dried rosemary, 1/2 teaspoon of sea salt, and 1/4 teaspoon of ground black pepper.

7. Cook the mixture for an additional 5 minutes, stirring occasionally, until everything is well combined and heated through.

8. Divide the hash among four plates and serve warm.

Nutritional Information (per serving):

- **Calories:** 250 kcal
- **Fat:** 10 grams (g) (Monounsaturated and polyunsaturated fats)
- **Carbohydrates:** 22 grams (g)
- **Proteins:** 18 grams (g)

<u>Coconut Yogurt Parfait with Mixed Berries and Flax Seeds</u>

Prep Time: 10 minutes | **Cook Time:** 0 minutes | **Servings:** 4

Ingredients:

- 2 cups coconut yogurt
- 1 cup fresh strawberries, sliced
- 1 cup fresh blueberries
- 1 cup fresh raspberries
- 2 tablespoons flax seeds
- 2 tablespoons unsweetened shredded coconut

Instructions:

1. Wash the fresh strawberries, fresh blueberries, and fresh raspberries. Slice the fresh strawberries.
2. In four serving glasses or bowls, start by spooning 1/2 cup of coconut yogurt into each glass.
3. Divide the sliced strawberries, fresh blueberries, and fresh raspberries evenly among the four glasses, layering them on top of the coconut yogurt.
4. Sprinkle 1/2 tablespoon of flax seeds over the berries in each glass.
5. Finish by sprinkling 1/2 tablespoon of unsweetened shredded coconut on top of each parfait.
6. Serve immediately, or refrigerate until ready to serve.

Nutritional Information (per serving):

- **Calories:** 180 kcal
- **Fat:** 12 grams (g) (Monounsaturated and polyunsaturated fats)
- **Carbohydrates:** 15 grams (g)
- **Proteins:** 4 grams (g)

Scrambled Eggs with Sautéed Mushrooms and Kale

Prep Time: 10 minutes | **Cook Time:** 10 minutes | **Servings:** 4

Ingredients:

- 8 large eggs
- 1 cup fresh kale, chopped
- 1 cup mushrooms, sliced
- 1 small onion, diced
- 2 tablespoons olive oil
- 1/2 teaspoon sea salt
- 1/4 teaspoon ground black pepper

Instructions:

1. Wash and chop the fresh kale, slice the mushrooms, and dice the small onion.
2. In a large skillet, heat the olive oil over medium heat.
3. Add the diced onion to the skillet and sauté for about 3 minutes or until it becomes translucent. Add the sliced mushrooms and continue to sauté for another 4 minutes or until the mushrooms are tender. Add the chopped kale and cook for an additional 2 minutes, stirring occasionally.
4. While the vegetables are cooking, crack the eggs into a bowl, add the sea salt and ground black pepper, and beat them well.
5. Pour the beaten eggs into the skillet with the sautéed vegetables. Cook, stirring frequently, until the eggs are fully cooked and scrambled, about 3-4 minutes.
6. Divide the scrambled eggs and sautéed vegetables among four plates and serve warm.

Nutritional Information (per serving):

- **Calories:** 220 kcal
- **Fat:** 14 grams (g) (Monounsaturated and polyunsaturated fats)
- **Carbohydrates:** 6 grams (g)
- **Proteins:** 16 grams (g)

Banana and Almond Butter Smoothie

Prep Time: 5 minutes | **Cook Time:** 0 minutes | **Servings:** 2

Ingredients:

- 2 ripe bananas, sliced
- 2 tablespoons almond butter
- 1 cup unsweetened almond milk
- 1/2 teaspoon vanilla extract
- 1 tablespoon ground flax seeds
- 1 cup ice cubes

Instructions:

1. Slice the ripe bananas.
2. In a blender, combine the sliced bananas, almond butter, unsweetened almond milk, vanilla extract, ground flax seeds, and ice cubes.
3. Blend on high until the mixture is smooth and creamy.
4. Pour the smoothie into two glasses and serve immediately.

Nutritional Information (per serving):

- **Calories:** 220 kcal
- **Fat:** 11 grams (g) (Monounsaturated and polyunsaturated fats)
- **Carbohydrates:** 27 grams (g)
- **Proteins:** 5 grams (g)

Chia Seed Pudding with Mango and Blueberries

Prep Time: 10 minutes | **Cook Time:** 0 minutes (plus 4 hours refrigeration) | **Servings:** 4

Ingredients:

- 1/2 cup chia seeds

- 2 cups unsweetened coconut milk

- 1 teaspoon vanilla extract

- 1 tablespoon maple syrup (optional, based on individual reintroduction tolerance)

- 1 ripe mango, diced

- 1 cup fresh blueberries

Instructions:

1. In a medium bowl, whisk together the chia seeds, unsweetened coconut milk, vanilla extract, and maple syrup (if using).

2. Cover the bowl and refrigerate for at least 4 hours, or overnight, until the chia seeds have absorbed the liquid and the mixture has thickened to a pudding-like consistency.

3. Peel and dice the ripe mango.

4. Divide the chia pudding evenly into four serving bowls. Top each serving with the diced mango and fresh blueberries.

5. Serve immediately, or keep refrigerated until ready to serve.

Nutritional Information (per serving):

- **Calories:** 180 kcal

- **Fat:** 9 grams (g) (Monounsaturated and polyunsaturated fats)

- **Carbohydrates:** 22 grams (g)

- **Proteins:** 5 grams (g)

<u>Cassava Flour Pancakes with Maple Syrup and Strawberries</u>

Prep Time: 10 minutes | **Cook Time:** 15 minutes | **Servings:** 4

Ingredients:

- 1 cup cassava flour
- 1/2 teaspoon baking soda
- 1/4 teaspoon sea salt
- 1 cup unsweetened coconut milk
- 2 large eggs
- 1 tablespoon olive oil
- 1 teaspoon vanilla extract
- 1 tablespoon maple syrup (optional, based on individual reintroduction tolerance)
- 1 cup fresh strawberries, sliced
- Additional maple syrup for serving (optional, based on individual reintroduction tolerance)

Instructions:

1. In a large bowl, whisk together the cassava flour, baking soda, and sea salt.

2. In another bowl, mix the unsweetened coconut milk, large eggs, olive oil, vanilla extract, and 1 tablespoon of maple syrup (if using).

3. Pour the wet ingredients into the bowl with the dry ingredients. Stir until the batter is smooth and well combined.

4. Heat a non-stick skillet or griddle over medium heat. Lightly grease with a small amount of olive oil if needed.

5. Pour about 1/4 cup of batter onto the skillet for each pancake. Cook for 2-3 minutes until bubbles form on the surface. Flip and cook for an additional 2-3 minutes until golden brown and cooked through.

6. Stack the pancakes on four plates. Top with the sliced fresh strawberries. Drizzle with additional maple syrup if using.

Nutritional Information (per serving):

- **Calories:** 220 kcal
- **Fat:** 10 grams (g) (Monounsaturated and polyunsaturated fats)
- **Carbohydrates:** 28 grams (g)
- **Proteins:** 6 grams (g)

Breakfast Sausage Patties with Apple Slices

Prep Time: 15 minutes | **Cook Time:** 15 minutes | **Servings:** 4

Ingredients:

- 1-pound ground turkey
- 1 small apple, peeled and grated
- 1 small onion, finely diced
- 1 teaspoon dried sage
- 1 teaspoon dried thyme
- 1/2 teaspoon sea salt
- 1/4 teaspoon ground black pepper
- 2 tablespoons olive oil
- 1 large apple, sliced

Instructions:

1. In a large bowl, combine the ground turkey, peeled and grated small apple, finely diced small onion, dried sage, dried thyme, sea salt, and ground black pepper. Mix until all ingredients are well incorporated.

2. Divide the mixture into 8 equal portions and shape them into patties.

3. In a large skillet, heat the olive oil over medium heat.

4. Add the sausage patties to the skillet and cook for about 4-5 minutes on each side, or until they are browned and cooked through.

5. While the patties are cooking, wash and slice the large apple.

6. Arrange the cooked sausage patties on four plates. Serve each portion with fresh apple slices on the side.

Nutritional Information (per serving):

- **Calories:** 250 kcal
- **Fat:** 14 grams (g) (Monounsaturated and polyunsaturated fats)
- **Carbohydrates:** 12 grams (g)
- **Proteins:** 20 grams (g)

<u>Avocado Toast on AIP Bread with Soft-Boiled Eggs</u>

Prep Time: 10 minutes | **Cook Time:** 10 minutes | **Servings:** 4

Ingredients:

- 4 slices AIP-compliant bread
- 2 ripe avocados, peeled and mashed
- 1 teaspoon lemon juice
- 1/2 teaspoon sea salt
- 1/4 teaspoon ground black pepper
- 4 large eggs
- 1 tablespoon olive oil

Instructions:

1. Bring a pot of water to a boil. Gently add the large eggs and boil for 6-7 minutes for soft-boiled eggs. Take out the eggs and place them in a bowl of cold water to cool. Once cooled, peel the eggs.

2. Lightly brush the AIP-compliant bread slices with olive oil. Toast the bread in a skillet over medium heat until golden brown, or use a toaster.

3. In a bowl, mash the peeled avocados. Add the lemon juice, sea salt, and ground black pepper, and mix adequately.

4. Spread the mashed avocado mixture evenly over each slice of toasted AIP-compliant bread.

5. Slice the soft-boiled eggs in half and place two halves on top of each avocado toast.

6. Serve immediately, garnished with additional ground black pepper if desired.

Nutritional Information (per serving):

- **Calories:** 250 kcal
- **Fat:** 18 grams (g) (Monounsaturated and polyunsaturated fats)
- **Carbohydrates:** 14 grams (g)
- **Proteins:** 10 grams (g)

Green Smoothie Bowl with Hemp Seeds and Kiwi

Prep Time: 10 minutes | **Cook Time:** 0 minutes | **Servings:** 2

Ingredients:

- 2 cups fresh spinach
- 1 ripe banana, sliced
- 1 cup unsweetened coconut milk
- 1/2 avocado, peeled and diced
- 1 tablespoon hemp seeds
- 1 teaspoon vanilla extract
- 1 cup ice cubes
- 1 kiwi, peeled and sliced
- 2 tablespoons hemp seeds (for topping)

Instructions:

1. Slice the ripe banana and dice the peeled avocado.
2. In a blender, combine the fresh spinach, sliced banana, unsweetened coconut milk, diced avocado, 1 tablespoon of hemp seeds, vanilla extract, and ice cubes. Blend until smooth and creamy.
3. Divide the smoothie evenly into two bowls.
4. Top each smoothie bowl with sliced kiwi and 1 tablespoon of hemp seeds.
5. Serve immediately.

Nutritional Information (per serving):

- **Calories:** 220 kcal
- **Fat:** 13 grams (g) (Monounsaturated and polyunsaturated fats)
- **Carbohydrates:** 18 grams (g)
- **Proteins:** 7 grams (g)

Butternut Squash and Apple Breakfast Bake

Prep Time: 15 minutes | **Cook Time:** 45 minutes | **Servings:** 4

Ingredients:

- 1 medium butternut squash, peeled and diced
- 2 large apples, peeled and diced
- 1 small onion, diced
- 2 tablespoons olive oil
- 1 teaspoon dried thyme
- 1 teaspoon dried sage
- 1/2 teaspoon sea salt
- 1/4 teaspoon ground black pepper
- 4 large eggs

Instructions:

1. Peel and dice the medium butternut squash and large apples. Dice the small onion.

2. Preheat the oven to 375 degrees Fahrenheit (190 degrees Celsius).

3. In a large mixing bowl, combine the diced butternut squash, diced apples, and diced onion. Add the olive oil, dried thyme, dried sage, sea salt, and ground black pepper. Toss to coat evenly.

4. Spread the mixture evenly in a large baking dish. Bake in the preheated oven for 35-40 minutes, or until the butternut squash is tender.

5. Take out the baking dish from the oven. Make four small wells in the baked mixture and crack one large egg into each well.

6. Return the baking dish to the oven and bake for an additional 5-7 minutes, or until the eggs are set to your liking.

7. Divide the bake into four portions and serve warm.

Nutritional Information (per serving):

- **Calories:** 220 kcal
- **Fat:** 12 grams (g) (Monounsaturated and polyunsaturated fats)
- **Carbohydrates:** 20 grams (g)
- **Proteins:** 8 grams (g)

Smoked Salmon and Cucumber Salad

Prep Time: 15 minutes | **Cook Time:** 0 minutes | **Servings:** 2

Ingredients:

- 4 ounces smoked salmon, thinly sliced
- 1 cucumber, thinly sliced
- 1/2 small red onion, thinly sliced
- 1/4 cup fresh dill, chopped
- 1 tablespoon capers, drained
- 2 tablespoons olive oil
- 1 tablespoon lemon juice
- Sea salt, to taste
- Ground black pepper, to taste

Instructions:

1. Thinly slice the smoked salmon, cucumber, and red onion. Chop the fresh dill.
2. In a large bowl, combine the sliced smoked salmon, sliced cucumber, sliced red onion, chopped fresh dill, and drained capers.
3. In a small bowl, whisk together the olive oil and lemon juice. Season with sea salt and ground black pepper to taste.
4. Drizzle the dressing over the salad ingredients in the large bowl. Gently toss to coat everything evenly.
5. Divide the salad into two portions and serve immediately.

Nutritional Information (per serving):

- **Calories:** 250 kcal
- **Fat:** 18 grams (g) (Monounsaturated and polyunsaturated fats)
- **Carbohydrates:** 6 grams (g)
- **Proteins:** 18 grams (g)

Zucchini Noodles with Poached Eggs and Avocado

Prep Time: 15 minutes | **Cook Time:** 10 minutes | **Servings:** 2

Ingredients:

- 2 medium zucchinis
- 2 large eggs
- 1 avocado, sliced
- 1 tablespoon olive oil
- 1 tablespoon lemon juice
- Sea salt, to taste
- Ground black pepper, to taste
- Red pepper flakes, optional, for garnish
- Fresh basil leaves, for garnish

Instructions:

1. Using a spiralizer, spiralize the zucchinis into noodles. Alternatively, you can use a vegetable peeler to create long, thin strips resembling noodles.

2. In a medium pot, bring water to a gentle simmer. Crack each egg into a small bowl or cup, then gently slide them into the simmering water, one at a time. Poach for about 3-4 minutes until the egg whites are set but the yolks are still runny. Remove with a slotted spoon and set aside.

3. Heat olive oil in a large skillet over medium heat. Add the zucchini noodles and sauté for 2-3 minutes until just tender. Remove from heat.

4. Divide the zucchini noodles between two plates. Top each plate with sliced avocado and one poached egg.

5. Drizzle with lemon juice. Season with sea salt, ground black pepper, and red pepper flakes (if using). Garnish with fresh basil leaves.

6. Serve immediately while the poached eggs are warm.

Nutritional Information (per serving):

- **Calories:** 280 kcal
- **Fat:** 20 grams (g) (Monounsaturated and polyunsaturated fats)
- **Carbohydrates:** 15 grams (g)
- **Proteins:** 12 grams (g)

Lunch Recipes

Grilled Chicken Salad with Mixed Greens and Citrus Vinaigrette

Prep Time: 20 minutes | **Cook Time:** 15 minutes | **Servings:** 4

Ingredients:

- 1-pound boneless, skinless chicken breasts
- 6 cups mixed greens (such as spinach, arugula, and romaine)
- 1 cup cherry tomatoes, halved
- 1 cucumber, sliced
- 1/4 red onion, thinly sliced
- 1 avocado, sliced
- 1/4 cup fresh cilantro leaves
- 1/4 cup fresh parsley leaves

For the Citrus Vinaigrette:

- 1/4 cup freshly squeezed orange juice
- 2 tablespoons freshly squeezed lemon juice
- 1 tablespoon honey (optional, omit for strict AIP)
- 1 teaspoon Dijon mustard
- 1/4 cup extra virgin olive oil
- Salt and pepper to taste

Instructions:

1. Preheat the grill to medium-high heat.
2. Season the chicken breasts with salt and pepper. Grill for about 6-7 minutes per side, or until cooked through and no longer pink in the center. Remove from heat and let rest for 5 minutes before slicing.
3. In a large bowl, combine the mixed greens, cherry tomatoes, cucumber, red onion, avocado, cilantro, and parsley.
4. To make the citrus vinaigrette, whisk together orange juice, lemon juice, honey (if using), Dijon mustard, and olive oil until well combined. Season with salt and pepper to taste.
5. Pour the vinaigrette over the salad and toss gently to coat.
6. Divide the salad among plates and top with sliced grilled chicken.
7. Serve immediately.

Nutritional Information (per serving):

- **Calories:** 320 kcal
- **Fat:** 18g
- **Carbohydrates:** 12g
- **Proteins:** 28g

Turkey and Cranberry Lettuce Wraps with Pumpkin Seeds Vinaigrette

Prep Time: 20 minutes | **Cook Time:** 10 minutes | **Servings:** 4

Ingredients:

- 1-pound ground turkey
- 1 tablespoon olive oil
- 1/2 teaspoon ground sage
- 1/2 teaspoon dried thyme

- Salt and pepper to taste
- 8 large lettuce leaves (such as butter or romaine)
- 1/2 cup dried cranberries
- 1/4 cup pumpkin seeds

For the Pumpkin Seeds Vinaigrette:

- 1/4 cup pumpkin seed oil
- 2 tablespoons apple cider vinegar
- 1 tablespoon honey (optional, omit for strict AIP)

- 1/2 teaspoon ground mustard
- Salt and pepper to taste

Instructions:

1. In a large skillet, heat olive oil over medium-high heat. Add ground turkey, sage, thyme, salt, and pepper. Cook, breaking up the turkey with a spatula, until browned and cooked through, about 7-8 minutes. Remove from heat and set aside.

2. Wash and dry lettuce leaves. Arrange them on a serving platter.

3. In a small bowl, combine dried cranberries and pumpkin seeds.

4. To make the pumpkin seeds vinaigrette, whisk together pumpkin seed oil, apple cider vinegar, honey (if using), ground mustard, salt, and pepper until well combined.

5. Divide the cooked ground turkey among the lettuce leaves.

6. Sprinkle each wrap with the cranberry and pumpkin seed mixture.

7. Drizzle the pumpkin seeds vinaigrette over the wraps.

8. Serve immediately.

Nutritional Information (per serving):

- **Calories:** 320 kcal
- **Fat:** 20g
- **Carbohydrates:** 15g
- **Proteins:** 25g

<u>Shrimp and Avocado Salad with Lime Dressing</u>

Prep Time: 15 minutes | **Cook Time:** 5 minutes | **Servings:** 4

Ingredients:

- 1-pound medium shrimp, peeled and deveined
- 2 avocados, diced
- 4 cups mixed salad greens (such as baby spinach and arugula)
- 1/2 cup cherry tomatoes, halved
- 1/4 cup red onion, thinly sliced
- 1/4 cup fresh cilantro leaves

For the Lime Dressing:

- Juice of 2 limes
- 1/4 cup extra virgin olive oil
- 1 teaspoon honey (optional, omit for strict AIP)
- 1 garlic clove, minced
- Salt and pepper to taste

Instructions:

1. In a large skillet, heat olive oil over medium-high heat. Add shrimp and cook for about 2-3 minutes per side, or until pink and cooked through. Remove from heat and set aside.

2. In a large bowl, combine salad greens, diced avocado, cherry tomatoes, red onion, and fresh cilantro leaves.

3. To make the lime dressing, whisk together lime juice, olive oil, honey (if using), minced garlic, salt, and pepper until well combined.

4. Pour the lime dressing over the salad and toss gently to coat.

5. Divide the salad among plates and top each serving with cooked shrimp.

6. Serve immediately.

Nutritional Information (per serving):

- **Calories:** 290 kcal
- **Fat:** 20g
- **Carbohydrates:** 12g
- **Proteins:** 18g

Beef and Broccoli Stir-fry with Coconut Aminos and Cashews

Prep Time: 15 minutes | **Cook Time:** 15 minutes | **Servings:** 4

Ingredients:

- 1-pound flank steak, thinly sliced
- 2 cups broccoli florets
- 1 red bell pepper, thinly sliced
- 1/2 cup unsalted cashews
- 4 green onions, sliced

For the Stir-fry Sauce:

- 1/4 cup coconut aminos
- 2 tablespoons sesame oil
- 1 tablespoon honey (optional, omit for strict AIP)
- 1 garlic clove, minced
- 1 teaspoon grated fresh ginger
- 1 tablespoon arrowroot powder (optional, for thickening)
- Salt and pepper to taste

Instructions:

1. In a small bowl, whisk together coconut aminos, sesame oil, honey (if using), minced garlic, grated ginger, arrowroot powder (if using), salt, and pepper to make the stir-fry sauce. Set aside.

2. Heat a large skillet or wok over medium-high heat. Add the thinly sliced flank steak and cook for about 2-3 minutes until browned. Remove from skillet and set aside.

3. In the same skillet, add broccoli florets and red bell pepper. Stir-fry for about 3-4 minutes until vegetables are tender-crisp.

4. Return the cooked beef to the skillet. Pour the stir-fry sauce over the beef and vegetables. Cook for an additional 1-2 minutes until everything is heated through and sauce has thickened slightly.

5. Stir in unsalted cashews and sliced green onions. Cook for another minute.

6. Remove from heat and serve immediately.

Nutritional Information (per serving):

- **Calories:** 380 kcal
- **Fat:** 22g
- **Carbohydrates:** 14g
- **Proteins:** 30g

AIP Caesar Salad with Homemade Dressing and Sardines

Prep Time: 15 minutes | **Cook Time:** 0 minutes | **Servings:** 4

Ingredients:

- 2 cans (3.75 oz each) boneless, skinless sardines in olive oil
- 8 cups mixed salad greens (such as romaine lettuce and kale)
- 1/4 cup pumpkin seeds
- 1/4 cup nutritional yeast
- 1/4 cup extra virgin olive oil
- Juice of 1 lemon
- 1 garlic clove, minced
- 1/2 teaspoon Dijon mustard
- Salt and pepper to taste

Instructions:

1. In a large bowl, combine mixed salad greens and pumpkin seeds.

2. Drain the olive oil from the sardines into a small bowl. Mash the sardines with a fork and add them to the salad greens.

3. To make the dressing, whisk together nutritional yeast, extra virgin olive oil, lemon juice, minced garlic, Dijon mustard, salt, and pepper until well combined.

4. Pour the dressing over the salad and toss gently to coat evenly.

5. Divide the salad among plates and top each serving with sardines.

6. Serve immediately.

Nutritional Information (per serving):

- **Calories:** 320 kcal
- **Fat:** 25g
- **Carbohydrates:** 8g
- **Proteins:** 20g

Tuna Salad with Cucumber, Dill, and Lemon

Prep Time: 15 minutes | **Cook Time:** 0 minutes | **Servings:** 4

Ingredients:

- 2 cans (5 oz each) tuna, drained
- 1 cucumber, diced
- 1/4 cup fresh dill, chopped
- 1/4 cup red onion, finely chopped
- Juice of 1 lemon
- 1/4 cup extra virgin olive oil
- Salt and pepper to taste

Instructions:

1. In a large bowl, combine drained tuna, diced cucumber, chopped dill, and finely chopped red onion.
2. In a small bowl, whisk together lemon juice, extra virgin olive oil, salt, and pepper.
3. Pour the dressing over the tuna mixture in the large bowl.
4. Toss gently to combine all ingredients evenly.
5. Divide the tuna salad among plates and serve immediately.

Nutritional Information (per serving):

- **Calories:** 250 kcal
- **Fat:** 15g
- **Carbohydrates:** 4g
- **Proteins:** 25g

Roasted Vegetable and Quinoa Salad with Chicken

Prep Time: 20 minutes | **Cook Time:** 30 minutes | **Servings:** 4

Ingredients:

- 1-pound boneless, skinless chicken breasts
- 1 cup quinoa, rinsed
- 2 cups mixed vegetables (such as bell peppers, zucchini, and carrots), diced
- 1 red onion, sliced
- 2 tablespoons olive oil
- Salt and pepper to taste
- 4 cups mixed salad greens (such as baby spinach and arugula)
- 1/4 cup fresh parsley, chopped
- 1/4 cup fresh basil, chopped

For the Dressing:

- Juice of 1 lemon
- 1/4 cup extra virgin olive oil
- 1 garlic clove, minced
- 1 teaspoon Dijon mustard
- Salt and pepper to taste

Instructions:

1. Preheat oven to 400°F (200°C).

2. Season chicken breasts with salt and pepper. Place on a baking sheet and roast in the oven for 20-25 minutes, or until cooked through and no longer pink in the center. Remove from oven and let rest for 5 minutes before slicing.

3. In a medium saucepan, bring 2 cups of water to a boil. Add rinsed quinoa, reduce heat to low, cover, and simmer for 15 minutes, or until quinoa is cooked and water is absorbed. Remove from heat and fluff with a fork.

4. In a large bowl, toss mixed vegetables and sliced red onion with olive oil, salt, and pepper. Spread on a baking sheet in a single layer and roast in the oven for 15-20 minutes, or until vegetables are tender and slightly caramelized.

5. In a small bowl, whisk together lemon juice, extra virgin olive oil, minced garlic, Dijon mustard, salt, and pepper to make the dressing.

6. In a large serving bowl, combine cooked quinoa, roasted vegetables, mixed salad greens, chopped parsley, and chopped basil.

7. Drizzle the dressing over the salad and toss gently to coat all ingredients evenly.

8. Divide the salad among plates and top each serving with sliced roasted chicken breasts.

9. Serve immediately.

Nutritional Information (per serving):

- **Calories:** 420 kcal
- **Fat:** 18g
- **Carbohydrates:** 30g
- **Proteins:** 32g

Mixed Greens Salad with Egg Yolks and Olive Oil Dressing

Prep Time: 15 minutes | **Cook Time:** 0 minutes | **Servings:** 4

Ingredients:

- 8 cups mixed salad greens (such as spinach, arugula, and romaine)
- 4 large eggs, yolks separated
- 1/4 cup extra virgin olive oil
- Juice of 1 lemon
- Salt and pepper to taste
- Optional: additional toppings such as cherry tomatoes, cucumber slices, or nuts/seeds

Instructions:

1. Wash and dry the mixed salad greens thoroughly. Place them in a large salad bowl.
2. Separate the egg yolks from the whites. Discard the whites or save for another use.
3. In a small bowl, whisk together the egg yolks, extra virgin olive oil, lemon juice, salt, and pepper until well combined.
4. Pour the dressing over the mixed salad greens.
5. Toss gently to coat the greens evenly with the dressing.
6. Optionally, add any additional toppings such as cherry tomatoes, cucumber slices, or nuts/seeds.
7. Divide the salad among plates and serve immediately.

Nutritional Information (per serving):

- **Calories:** 220 kcal
- **Fat:** 20g
- **Carbohydrates:** 5g
- **Proteins:** 6g

Grilled Salmon with Arugula, Pomegranate Seeds, and Almonds

Prep Time: 15 minutes | **Cook Time:** 10 minutes | **Servings:** 4

Ingredients:

- 4 salmon fillets, about 6 oz each
- Salt and pepper to taste
- 8 cups arugula
- 1/2 cup pomegranate seeds
- 1/4 cup almonds, sliced or chopped
- 1/4 cup extra virgin olive oil
- Juice of 1 lemon
- Optional: additional seasonings such as garlic powder or herbs

Instructions:

1. Preheat the grill to medium-high heat.
2. Season the salmon fillets with salt and pepper on both sides.
3. Place the salmon fillets on the preheated grill and cook for about 4-5 minutes per side, or until the salmon is cooked through and flakes easily with a fork.
4. While the salmon is grilling, prepare the salad. In a large salad bowl, combine arugula, pomegranate seeds, and sliced or chopped almonds.
5. In a small bowl, whisk together extra virgin olive oil, lemon juice, and any optional seasonings.
6. Pour the dressing over the arugula salad and toss gently to coat evenly.
7. Divide the dressed arugula salad among plates.
8. Place a grilled salmon fillet on top of each serving of salad.
9. Serve immediately.

Nutritional Information (per serving):

- **Calories:** 400 kcal
- **Fat:** 25g
- **Carbohydrates:** 10g
- **Proteins:** 30g

Turkey and Apple Slaw with Carrot-Ginger Dressing

Prep Time: 20 minutes | **Cook Time:** 0 minutes | **Servings:** 4

Ingredients:

- 1-pound cooked turkey breast, shredded
- 2 cups shredded green cabbage
- 1 apple, thinly sliced
- 1/2 cup shredded carrots
- 1/4 cup fresh cilantro, chopped
- 1/4 cup sliced almonds

For the Carrot-Ginger Dressing:

- 1/2 cup shredded carrots
- 1 tablespoon fresh ginger, grated
- Juice of 1 lemon
- 1/4 cup extra virgin olive oil
- Salt and pepper to taste

Instructions:

1. In a large bowl, combine shredded turkey breast, shredded green cabbage, thinly sliced apple, shredded carrots, chopped cilantro, and sliced almonds.
2. To make the carrot-ginger dressing, blend together shredded carrots, grated fresh ginger, lemon juice, extra virgin olive oil, salt, and pepper until smooth.
3. Pour the carrot-ginger dressing over the turkey and vegetable mixture in the bowl.
4. Toss gently to coat all ingredients evenly with the dressing.
5. Divide the turkey and apple slaw among plates.
6. Serve immediately.

Nutritional Information (per serving):

- **Calories:** 300 kcal
- **Fat:** 15g
- **Carbohydrates:** 15g
- **Proteins:** 25g

Zucchini Noodles with Walnut Pesto and Cherry Tomatoes

Prep Time: 20 minutes | **Cook Time:** 10 minutes | **Servings:** 4

Ingredients:

- 4 medium zucchinis
- 1 cup cherry tomatoes, halved
- 1/4 cup walnuts, chopped
- 1/4 cup fresh basil leaves
- 1/4 cup fresh parsley leaves
- 1/4 cup extra virgin olive oil
- Juice of 1 lemon
- 1 garlic clove, minced
- Salt and pepper to taste
- Optional: grated Parmesan cheese (for non-AIP version)

Instructions:

1. Using a spiralizer or a vegetable peeler, create zucchini noodles (zoodles) from the zucchinis. Set aside.

2. In a food processor, combine chopped walnuts, basil leaves, parsley leaves, extra virgin olive oil, lemon juice, minced garlic, salt, and pepper. Blend until the mixture forms a smooth pesto sauce.

3. In a large skillet, heat a small amount of olive oil over medium heat. Add cherry tomatoes and cook for 2-3 minutes, until slightly softened.

4. Add the zucchini noodles to the skillet with the cherry tomatoes. Cook for 3-4 minutes, tossing gently with tongs, until the zucchini noodles are just tender.

5. Take out the skillet from heat and stir in the walnut pesto sauce, tossing gently to coat the zucchini noodles and cherry tomatoes evenly.

6. Divide the zucchini noodles with walnut pesto and cherry tomatoes among plates.

7. Optional: Serve with grated Parmesan cheese for non-AIP version.

Nutritional Information (per serving):

- **Calories:** 250 kcal
- **Fat:** 20g
- **Carbohydrates:** 10g
- **Proteins:** 6g

Baked Cod with Spinach, Avocado Salsa, and Sweet Potatoes

Prep Time: 20 minutes | **Cook Time:** 25 minutes | **Servings:** 4

Ingredients:

- 4 cod fillets, about 6 oz each
- 2 sweet potatoes, peeled and diced
- 4 cups fresh spinach leaves
- 2 avocados, diced
- 1/2 red onion, finely chopped
- Juice of 1 lime
- 2 tablespoons extra virgin olive oil
- Salt and pepper to taste

Instructions:

1. Preheat the oven to 400°F (200°C).

2. Place the diced sweet potatoes on a baking sheet lined with parchment paper. Drizzle with 1 tablespoon of olive oil and season with salt and pepper. Toss to coat evenly. Bake in the preheated oven for 20-25 minutes, or until tender and lightly browned, stirring halfway through.

3. While the sweet potatoes are baking, prepare the avocado salsa. In a bowl, combine diced avocados, finely chopped red onion, lime juice, 1 tablespoon of olive oil, salt, and pepper. Toss gently to mix adequately. Set aside.

4. Season the cod fillets with salt and pepper on both sides.

5. Heat a non-stick skillet over medium heat. Add the cod fillets and cook for 2-3 minutes per side, until lightly browned.

6. Take out the cod fillets from the skillet and place them on a baking sheet lined with parchment paper.

7. Place the baking sheet with the cod fillets in the oven and bake for 8-10 minutes, or until the cod is cooked through and flakes easily with a fork.

8. While the cod is baking, wilt the spinach. In the same skillet used for the cod, add the spinach leaves and cook over medium heat for 2-3 minutes, stirring frequently, until wilted.

9. To serve, divide the baked sweet potatoes and wilted spinach among plates. Top each serving with a baked cod fillet and spoon the avocado salsa over the cod.

10. Serve immediately.

Nutritional Information (per serving):

- **Calories:** 400 kcal
- **Fat:** 20g
- **Carbohydrates:** 30g
- **Proteins:** 30g

Dinner Recipes

Herb-Roasted Chicken with Brussels Sprouts and Sweet Potato Mash

Prep Time: 15 minutes | **Cook Time:** 45 minutes | **Servings:** 4

Ingredients:

For Herb-Roasted Chicken:

- 4 boneless, skinless chicken breasts
- 2 tablespoons olive oil
- 2 cloves garlic, minced
- 1 teaspoon dried thyme
- 1 teaspoon dried rosemary
- Salt and pepper to taste

For Brussels Sprouts:

- 1-pound Brussels sprouts, trimmed and halved
- 1 tablespoon olive oil
- Salt and pepper to taste

For Sweet Potato Mash:

- 2 large sweet potatoes, peeled and cubed
- 1 tablespoon olive oil
- 1/4 cup unsweetened almond milk (or coconut milk for AIP)
- Salt to taste

Instructions:

1. Preheat your oven to 400°F (200°C).
2. In a small bowl, combine olive oil, minced garlic, dried thyme, dried rosemary, salt, and pepper.
3. Rub the mixture over the chicken breasts evenly.
4. Place the chicken breasts on a baking sheet lined with parchment paper.
5. Roast in the preheated oven for 25-30 minutes or until the chicken reaches an internal temperature of 165°F (74°C).
6. Toss the halved Brussels sprouts with olive oil, salt, and pepper on a separate baking sheet lined with parchment paper.
7. Place in the oven alongside the chicken and roast for 20-25 minutes until tender and lightly browned.
8. While the chicken and Brussels sprouts are roasting, boil the cubed sweet potatoes in a pot of water until fork-tender, about 10-15 minutes.
9. Drain the sweet potatoes and mash them with olive oil, almond milk (or coconut milk for AIP), and salt until smooth.
10. Divide the sweet potato mash among plates.
11. Slice the herb-roasted chicken and serve alongside the roasted Brussels sprouts.
12. Enjoy your Herb-Roasted Chicken with Brussels Sprouts and Sweet Potato Mash!

Nutritional Information (per serving):

- **Calories:** 380 kcal
- **Fat:** 14g
- **Carbohydrates:** 30g
- **Protein:** 32g

Baked Salmon with Asparagus and Lemon Dill Sauce Potato Mash

Prep Time: 15 minutes | **Cook Time:** 20 minutes | **Servings:** 4

Ingredients:

For Baked Salmon:

- 4 salmon fillets (about 6 ounces each)
- 2 tablespoons olive oil
- 2 cloves garlic, minced
- 1 teaspoon dried dill
- Salt and pepper to taste

For Asparagus:

- 1-pound asparagus, trimmed
- 1 tablespoon olive oil
- Salt and pepper to taste

For Lemon Dill Sauce:

- 1/2 cup unsweetened almond milk (or coconut milk for AIP)
- Juice of 1 lemon
- 1 teaspoon dried dill
- Salt and pepper to taste

For Potato Mash:

- 4 medium potatoes, peeled and cubed
- 1 tablespoon olive oil
- 1/4 cup unsweetened almond milk (or coconut milk for AIP)
- Salt to taste

Instructions:

1. Preheat your oven to 400°F (200°C).
2. In a small bowl, mix olive oil, minced garlic, dried dill, salt, and pepper.
3. Rub the mixture over the salmon fillets evenly.
4. Place the salmon fillets on a baking sheet lined with parchment paper.
5. Bake in the preheated oven for 15-20 minutes or until the salmon flakes easily with a fork.
6. Toss the trimmed asparagus with olive oil, salt, and pepper on a separate baking sheet lined with parchment paper.
7. Place in the oven alongside the salmon and roast for 10-12 minutes until tender-crisp.
8. In a small saucepan, heat almond milk (or coconut milk for AIP) over medium heat.
9. Stir in lemon juice, dried dill, salt, and pepper.
10. Simmer for 2-3 minutes until slightly thickened. Adjust seasoning to taste.
11. While the salmon and asparagus are baking, boil the cubed potatoes in a pot of water until fork-tender, about 10-15 minutes.
12. Drain the potatoes and mash them with olive oil, almond milk (or coconut milk for AIP), and salt until smooth. Next, divide the lemon dill sauce among plates.
13. Place a portion of the baked salmon and asparagus on each plate, and serve with a side of the mash.

Nutritional Information (per serving):

- **Calories:** 380 kcal
- **Fat:** 18g
- **Carbohydrates:** 30g
- **Protein:** 30g

Beef and Vegetable Stew with Root Vegetables Mash

Prep Time: 20 minutes | **Cook Time:** 2 hours | **Servings:** 6

Ingredients:

For Beef and Vegetable Stew:

- 1.5 pounds stewing beef, cubed
- 2 tablespoons olive oil
- 2 cloves garlic, minced
- 1 onion, chopped
- 2 carrots, peeled and diced
- 2 celery stalks, diced
- 1 parsnip, peeled and diced
- 1 turnip, peeled and diced
- 1 teaspoon dried thyme
- 1 teaspoon dried rosemary
- 4 cups beef broth (low sodium for AIP)
- Salt and pepper to taste

For Root Vegetables Mash:

- 2 large sweet potatoes, peeled and cubed
- 2 large carrots, peeled and cubed
- 1 medium parsnip, peeled and cubed
- 1 medium turnip, peeled and cubed
- 1 tablespoon olive oil
- 1/4 cup unsweetened almond milk (or coconut milk for AIP)
- Salt to taste

Instructions:

1. In a large pot, heat olive oil over medium-high heat.
2. Add cubed stewing beef and brown on all sides.
3. Add minced garlic, chopped onion, diced carrots, diced celery, diced parsnip, and diced turnip to the pot.
4. Cook for 5-7 minutes until vegetables start to soften.
5. Stir in dried thyme, dried rosemary, salt, and pepper.
6. Pour in beef broth, bring to a boil, then reduce heat to low.
7. Cover and simmer for 1.5 to 2 hours, stirring occasionally, until beef is tender and flavors are well blended.
8. While the stew is simmering, boil the cubed sweet potatoes, carrots, parsnip, and turnip in a pot of water until fork-tender, about 15-20 minutes.
9. Drain the vegetables and mash them with olive oil, almond milk (or coconut milk for AIP), and salt until smooth.
10. Divide the root vegetables mash among plates.
11. Ladle the beef and vegetable stew over the mash.
12. Garnish with fresh herbs if desired.
13. Enjoy your Beef and Vegetable Stew with Root Vegetables Mash!

Nutritional Information (per serving):

- **Calories:** 420 kcal
- **Fat:** 14g
- **Carbohydrates:** 38g
- **Protein:** 35g

Pork Tenderloin with Apple Compote and Roasted Carrots

Prep Time: 15 minutes | **Cook Time:** 30 minutes | **Servings:** 4

Ingredients:

For Pork Tenderloin:

- 1-pound pork tenderloin
- 2 tablespoons olive oil
- 2 cloves garlic, minced
- 1 teaspoon dried thyme
- Salt and pepper to taste

For Apple Compote:

- 2 apples, peeled, cored, and diced
- 1 tablespoon olive oil
-
- 1/4 cup unsweetened apple juice
- 1 teaspoon ground cinnamon

For Roasted Carrots:

- 1-pound carrots, peeled and cut into sticks
- 1 tablespoon olive oil
- Salt and pepper to taste

Instructions:

1. Preheat your oven to 400°F (200°C).
2. In a small bowl, mix olive oil, minced garlic, dried thyme, salt, and pepper.
3. Rub the mixture over the pork tenderloin evenly.
4. Heat an oven-safe skillet over medium-high heat.
5. Sear the pork tenderloin on all sides until browned, about 2-3 minutes per side.
6. Transfer the skillet with the pork tenderloin to the preheated oven.
7. Roast for 20-25 minutes or until the internal temperature reaches 145°F (63°C).
8. Remove from the oven and let it rest for 5 minutes before slicing.
9. While the pork is roasting, heat olive oil in a saucepan over medium heat.
10. Add diced apples and cook until softened, about 5 minutes.
11. Stir in unsweetened apple juice and ground cinnamon. Next, simmer for 5-7 minutes until the liquid has reduced and apples are tender. Remove from heat.
12. Toss carrot sticks with olive oil, salt, and pepper on a baking sheet lined with parchment paper.
13. Roast in the oven for 20-25 minutes, stirring halfway through, until carrots are tender and slightly caramelized. Next, slice the pork tenderloin and divide among plates.
14. Spoon apple compote over the pork slices.
15. Serve with roasted carrots on the side.
16. Enjoy your Pork Tenderloin with Apple Compote and Roasted Carrots!

Nutritional Information (per serving):

- **Calories:** 350 kcal
- **Fat:** 14g
- **Carbohydrates:** 20g
- **Protein:** 30g

Lemon-Garlic Shrimp with Zucchini Noodles and Pesto

Prep Time: 15 minutes | **Cook Time:** 10 minutes | **Servings:** 4

Ingredients:

For Lemon-Garlic Shrimp:

- 1-pound large shrimp, peeled and deveined
- 2 tablespoons olive oil
- 4 cloves garlic, minced
- Zest of 1 lemon
- Juice of 1 lemon
- Salt and pepper to taste

For Zucchini Noodles:

- 4 medium zucchini, spiralized into noodles
- 1 tablespoon olive oil
- Salt and pepper to taste

For Pesto:

- 1 cup fresh basil leaves
- 1/4 cup pine nuts
- 1/4 cup olive oil
- 2 cloves garlic, minced
- Salt and pepper to taste

Instructions:

1. In a food processor, combine basil leaves, pine nuts, olive oil, minced garlic, salt, and pepper.
2. Pulse until smooth. Adjust seasoning to taste. Set aside.
3. In a large skillet, heat olive oil over medium-high heat.
4. Add minced garlic and cook until fragrant, about 1 minute.
5. Add shrimp to the skillet, spreading them out in a single layer.
6. Cook for 2-3 minutes per side until shrimp are pink and cooked through.
7. Stir in lemon zest, lemon juice, salt, and pepper. Remove from heat.
8. In another skillet, heat olive oil over medium heat.
9. Add zucchini noodles and sauté for 2-3 minutes until just tender.
10. Season with salt and pepper to taste.
11. Divide the zucchini noodles among plates.
12. Top with lemon-garlic shrimp.
13. Drizzle pesto over the shrimp and noodles.
14. Garnish with additional basil leaves if desired.
15. Enjoy your Lemon-Garlic Shrimp with Zucchini Noodles and Pesto!

Nutritional Information (per serving):

- **Calories:** 320 kcal
- **Fat:** 18g
- **Carbohydrates:** 10g
- **Protein:** 30g

Lamb Chops with Mint, Roasted Root Vegetables, and Pomegranate Seeds

Prep Time: 20 minutes | **Cook Time:** 40 minutes | **Servings:** 4

Ingredients:

For Lamb Chops:

- 8 lamb loin chops
- 2 tablespoons olive oil
- 2 cloves garlic, minced
- 2 tablespoons fresh mint leaves, chopped
- Salt and pepper to taste

For Roasted Root Vegetables:

- 2 large carrots, peeled and cut into chunks
- 2 parsnips, peeled and cut into chunks
- 1 sweet potato, peeled and cut into chunks
- 1 turnip, peeled and cut into chunks
- 2 tablespoons olive oil
- Salt and pepper to taste

For Garnish:

- 1/2 cup pomegranate seeds
- Fresh mint leaves for garnish

Instructions:

1. Preheat your oven to 400°F (200°C).
2. In a small bowl, mix olive oil, minced garlic, chopped mint leaves, salt, and pepper.
3. Rub the mixture over the lamb chops evenly.
4. Heat a large oven-safe skillet over medium-high heat.
5. Sear the lamb chops for 2-3 minutes per side until browned.
6. Transfer the skillet with the lamb chops to the preheated oven.
7. Roast for 10-15 minutes for medium-rare, or longer according to desired doneness.
8. Toss carrot chunks, parsnip chunks, sweet potato chunks, and turnip chunks with olive oil, salt, and pepper on a baking sheet lined with parchment paper.
9. Roast in the oven for 25-30 minutes, stirring halfway through, until vegetables are tender and golden brown.
10. Arrange roasted root vegetables on a serving platter.
11. Place the lamb chops on top of the vegetables.
12. Sprinkle with pomegranate seeds and garnish with fresh mint leaves.
13. Enjoy your Lamb Chops with Mint, Roasted Root Vegetables, and Pomegranate Seeds!

Nutritional Information (per serving):

- **Calories:** 450 kcal
- **Fat:** 26g
- **Carbohydrates:** 20g
- **Protein:** 32g

Grilled Steak with Chimichurri Sauce and Cauliflower Rice

Prep Time: 15 minutes | **Cook Time:** 15 minutes | **Servings:** 4

Ingredients:

For Grilled Steak:

- 4 steaks of your choice (such as sirloin, ribeye, or flank steak), about 6 ounces each
- 2 tablespoons olive oil
- 2 cloves garlic, minced
- 1 teaspoon dried oregano
- Salt and pepper to taste

For Chimichurri Sauce:

- 1 cup fresh parsley leaves, chopped
- 1/4 cup fresh cilantro leaves, chopped
- 2 cloves garlic, minced
- 1/4 cup red wine vinegar
- 1/2 cup olive oil
- Salt and pepper to taste

For Cauliflower Rice:

- 1 large head of cauliflower, grated or processed into rice-sized pieces
- 2 tablespoons olive oil
- Salt and pepper to taste

Instructions:

1. In a bowl, combine chopped parsley, chopped cilantro, minced garlic, red wine vinegar, olive oil, salt, and pepper.
2. Mix adequately and set aside to let flavors meld.
3. In a small bowl, mix olive oil, minced garlic, dried oregano, salt, and pepper.
4. Rub the mixture over the steaks evenly.
5. Preheat grill or grill pan to medium-high heat.
6. Grill steaks for 4-6 minutes per side, or until desired doneness is reached.
7. Remove from grill and let rest for 5 minutes before slicing.
8. Heat olive oil in a large skillet over medium heat.
9. Add cauliflower rice and sauté for 5-7 minutes until tender.
10. Season with salt and pepper to taste.
11. Divide cauliflower rice among plates.
12. Slice grilled steaks and place on top of cauliflower rice.
13. Drizzle chimichurri sauce over the steaks.
14. Garnish with additional parsley or cilantro if desired.
15. Enjoy your Grilled Steak with Chimichurri Sauce and Cauliflower Rice!

Nutritional Information (per serving):

- **Calories:** 450 kcal
- **Fat:** 28g
- **Carbohydrates:** 10g
- **Protein:** 40g

Coconut Chicken Curry with Cauliflower Rice and Spinach

Prep Time: 15 minutes | **Cook Time:** 25 minutes | **Servings:** 4

Ingredients:

For Coconut Chicken Curry:

- 1-pound boneless, skinless chicken breasts, cut into bite-sized pieces
- 2 tablespoons coconut oil
- 1 onion, finely chopped
- 3 cloves garlic, minced
- 1 tablespoon fresh ginger, grated
- 1 tablespoon curry powder
- 1 teaspoon ground turmeric
- 1 can (14 oz) coconut milk (full-fat for AIP)
- 1 cup chicken broth (low sodium for AIP)
- Salt and pepper to taste
- Fresh cilantro for garnish

For Cauliflower Rice:

- 1 large head of cauliflower, grated or processed into rice-sized pieces
- 2 tablespoons coconut oil
- Salt to taste

For Spinach:

- 4 cups fresh spinach leaves
- 1 tablespoon coconut oil
- Salt and pepper to taste

Instructions:

1. In a large skillet, heat coconut oil over medium-high heat.
2. Add chopped onion and sauté until translucent, about 3-4 minutes.
3. Add minced garlic and grated ginger, and cook for 1 minute until fragrant.
4. Add curry powder and ground turmeric, stir to coat the onion mixture.
5. Add chicken pieces to the skillet and cook until chicken is browned on all sides, about 5-7 minutes.
6. Pour in coconut milk and chicken broth, stir to combine. Bring to a boil, then reduce heat to low. Next, simmer uncovered for 10-15 minutes until chicken is cooked through and sauce is slightly thickened. Season with salt and pepper to taste.
7. Heat coconut oil in a large skillet over medium heat.
8. Add cauliflower rice and sauté for 5-7 minutes until tender. Season with salt to taste.
9. In a separate skillet, heat coconut oil over medium heat.
10. Add spinach leaves and sauté until wilted, about 2-3 minutes. Season with salt and pepper to taste. Next, divide cauliflower rice among plates.
11. Spoon coconut chicken curry over the cauliflower rice.
12. Serve with sautéed spinach on the side. Garnish with fresh cilantro.

Nutritional Information (per serving):

- **Calories:** 380 kcal
- **Protein:** 30g
- **Fat:** 25g
- **Carbohydrates:** 10g

AIP Meatloaf with Mashed Parsnips and Green Beans

Prep Time: 20 minutes | **Cook Time:** 1 hour | **Servings:** 4

Ingredients:

For AIP Meatloaf:

- 1-pound ground beef (preferably grass-fed)
- 1 onion, finely chopped
- 2 cloves garlic, minced
- 1/2 cup chopped fresh parsley
- 1/4 cup chopped fresh basil
- 1/4 cup chopped fresh cilantro
- 1 teaspoon dried oregano
- Salt and pepper to taste
- 1/4 cup coconut flour
- 1/4 cup coconut milk (full-fat, AIP compliant)

For Mashed Parsnips:

- 4 large parsnips, peeled and chopped
- 2 tablespoons coconut oil
- Salt to taste

For Green Beans:

- 1-pound fresh green beans, trimmed
- 2 tablespoons olive oil
- Salt and pepper to taste

Instructions:

1. Preheat oven to 375°F (190°C).
2. In a large bowl, combine ground beef, chopped onion, minced garlic, chopped parsley, basil, cilantro, dried oregano, salt, pepper, coconut flour, and coconut milk.
3. Mix until well combined. Transfer mixture to a loaf pan and press down evenly.
4. Bake for 45-50 minutes until cooked through and browned on top.
5. While the meatloaf is baking, place chopped parsnips in a pot and cover with water.
6. Bring to a boil over medium-high heat, then reduce to a simmer.
7. Cook for 15-20 minutes until parsnips are tender.
8. Drain parsnips and transfer to a food processor. Next, add coconut oil and salt, then process until smooth and creamy. Adjust seasoning if needed.
9. Steam or boil green beans until tender-crisp, about 4-5 minutes.
10. Drain and toss with olive oil, salt, and pepper.
11. Slice AIP Meatloaf and serve alongside mashed parsnips and green beans.

Nutritional Information (per serving):

- **Calories:** 450 kcal
- **Fat:** 28g
- **Carbohydrates:** 25g
- **Protein:** 30g

Ginger-Turmeric Chicken Thighs with Roasted Broccoli

Prep Time: 15 minutes | **Cook Time:** 25 minutes | **Servings:** 4

Ingredients:

For Ginger-Turmeric Chicken Thighs:

- 4 bone-in, skin-on chicken thighs
- 2 tablespoons olive oil
- 1 tablespoon fresh ginger, grated
- 1 tablespoon ground turmeric
- 2 cloves garlic, minced
- Salt and pepper to taste

For Roasted Broccoli:

- 1 large head of broccoli, cut into florets
- 2 tablespoons olive oil
- Salt and pepper to taste

Instructions:

1. Preheat your oven to 400°F (200°C).
2. In a small bowl, mix olive oil, grated ginger, ground turmeric, minced garlic, salt, and pepper.
3. Rub the mixture over the chicken thighs evenly, ensuring they are well coated.
4. Place the chicken thighs skin-side up on a baking sheet lined with parchment paper.
5. Roast in the preheated oven for 20-25 minutes, or until the chicken reaches an internal temperature of 165°F (74°C) and the skin is crispy.
6. While the chicken is roasting, toss broccoli florets with olive oil, salt, and pepper on another baking sheet lined with parchment paper.
7. Spread the broccoli in a single layer.
8. Place the broccoli in the oven alongside the chicken during the last 15 minutes of cooking time.
9. Roast for 15 minutes, or until the broccoli is tender and lightly browned around the edges.
10. Take out the chicken thighs and broccoli from the oven.
11. Serve the Ginger-Turmeric Chicken Thighs with Roasted Broccoli hot.
12. Enjoy your flavorful and nutritious meal!

Nutritional Information (per serving):

- **Calories:** 380 kcal
- **Fat:** 25g
- **Carbohydrates:** 10g
- **Protein:** 30g

Baked Cod with Almond Crust, Green Beans, and Carrot Purée

Prep Time: 20 minutes | **Cook Time:** 20 minutes | **Servings:** 4

Ingredients:

For Baked Cod:

- 4 cod fillets (about 6 ounces each)
- 1/2 cup almond flour
- 1/2 cup almonds, finely chopped
- 1 teaspoon paprika
- 1/2 teaspoon garlic powder
- Salt and pepper to taste
- 2 tablespoons olive oil

For Green Beans:

- 1-pound fresh green beans, trimmed
- 2 tablespoons olive oil
- Salt and pepper to taste

For Carrot Purée:

- 4 large carrots, peeled and chopped
- 2 tablespoons coconut oil
- Salt and pepper to taste

Instructions:

1. Preheat your oven to 400°F (200°C).
2. In a shallow bowl, combine almond flour, chopped almonds, paprika, garlic powder, salt, and pepper. Pat dry the cod fillets with paper towels.
3. Brush each cod fillet with olive oil, then coat evenly with the almond mixture, pressing gently to adhere. Place the coated cod fillets on a baking sheet lined with parchment paper.
4. Bake in the preheated oven for 15-20 minutes, or until the cod is opaque and flakes easily with a fork.
5. While the cod is baking, toss green beans with olive oil, salt, and pepper on another baking sheet lined with parchment paper.
6. Spread the green beans in a single layer.
7. Place the green beans in the oven alongside the cod during the last 10-12 minutes of cooking time. Roast until the green beans are tender-crisp and slightly browned.
8. While the cod and green beans are roasting, place chopped carrots in a pot and cover with water.
9. Bring to a boil over medium-high heat, then reduce to a simmer.
10. Cook for 10-12 minutes until carrots are very tender.
11. Drain the carrots and transfer to a food processor.
12. Add coconut oil, salt, and pepper, then process until smooth and creamy.
13. Divide the carrot purée among plates.
14. Place a baked cod fillet on each plate.
15. Serve with roasted green beans on the side.

Nutritional Information (per serving):

- **Calories:** 380 kcal
- **Fat:** 22g
- **Carbohydrates:** 15g
- **Protein:** 30g

Stuffed Bell Peppers with Ground Beef, Quinoa, and Spinach

Prep Time: 30 minutes | **Cook Time:** 45 minutes | **Servings:** 6

Ingredients:

For Stuffed Bell Peppers:

- 6 large bell peppers, any color
- 1-pound lean ground beef
- 1 cup quinoa, cooked
- 1 onion, finely chopped
- 2 cloves garlic, minced
- 2 cups fresh spinach, chopped
- 1 can (14.5 ounces) diced tomatoes, drained
- 1 teaspoon dried oregano
- 1 teaspoon dried basil
- Salt and pepper to taste
- Olive oil, for cooking

Instructions:

1. Preheat your oven to 375°F (190°C).
2. Cut the tops off the bell peppers and take out the seeds and membranes.
3. Place the bell peppers in a baking dish, cut-side up.
4. Cook quinoa according to package instructions. Set aside.
5. In a large skillet, heat olive oil over medium heat.
6. Add chopped onion and garlic, sauté until softened.
7. Add ground beef to the skillet, cook until browned and no longer pink.
8. Drain any excess fat. Next, stir in chopped spinach, diced tomatoes, dried oregano, dried basil, cooked quinoa, salt, and pepper.
9. Cook for another 2-3 minutes until the spinach is wilted and the flavors are combined.
10. Spoon the beef and quinoa mixture evenly into each bell pepper.
11. Press down gently to pack the filling.
12. Cover the baking dish with foil and bake in the preheated oven for 30-35 minutes, or until the bell peppers are tender.
13. Remove from the oven and let cool slightly.
14. Serve the Stuffed Bell Peppers hot, optionally garnished with fresh herbs.
15. Enjoy your delicious and nutritious meal!

Nutritional Information (per serving):

- **Calories:** 320 kcal
- **Fat:** 12g
- **Carbohydrates:** 30g
- **Protein:** 24g

Snacks Recipes

Apple Slices with Almond Butter and Cinnamon

Prep Time: 10 minutes | **Cook Time:** 0 minutes | **Servings:** 2

Ingredients:

- 1 medium apple, sliced

- 4 tablespoons almond butter

- 1/2 teaspoon ground cinnamon

- Optional: drizzle of honey or maple syrup (avoid for strict AIP)

Instructions:

1. Wash and slice the apple into thin slices.

2. Spread 2 tablespoons of almond butter evenly over each apple slice.

3. Sprinkle ground cinnamon over the almond butter.

4. If using, drizzle honey or maple syrup over the apple slices (avoid for strict AIP).

5. Arrange the apple slices on a plate and enjoy immediately.

Nutritional Information per Serving:

- **Calories:** 220 kcal

- **Fat:** 14g

- **Carbohydrates:** 20g

- **Proteins:** 7g

Carrot and Celery Sticks with AIP Ranch Dip

Prep Time: 15 minutes | **Cook Time:** 0 minutes | **Servings:** 4

Ingredients:

- 2 large carrots, peeled and cut into sticks

- 4 celery stalks, cut into sticks

- **AIP Ranch Dip:**

  - 1/2 cup coconut milk (full-fat)
  - 2 tablespoons olive oil
  - 1 tablespoon apple cider vinegar
  - 1/2 teaspoon garlic powder
  - 1/2 teaspoon onion powder
  - 1/2 teaspoon dried parsley
  - 1/2 teaspoon dried dill
  - Salt, to taste

Instructions:

1. Wash, peel (if needed), and cut the carrots and celery into sticks.

2. **Make the AIP Ranch Dip:**

   - In a bowl, whisk together the coconut milk, olive oil, apple cider vinegar, garlic powder, onion powder, dried parsley, dried dill, and salt until well combined.

3. Arrange the carrot and celery sticks on a plate alongside the AIP Ranch Dip.

Nutritional Information per Serving:

- **Calories:** 130 kcal

- **Fat:** 11g

- **Carbohydrates:** 7g

- **Proteins:** 2g

Homemade AIP Granola Bars with Pumpkin Seeds and Coconut

Prep Time: 15 minutes | **Cook Time:** 25 minutes | **Servings:** 10 bars

Ingredients:

- 1 cup shredded coconut
- 1 cup pumpkin seeds
- 1/2 cup chopped dried apricots
- 1/2 cup chopped dates
- 1/4 cup melted coconut oil
- 1/4 cup honey or maple syrup (avoid for strict AIP)
- 1/2 teaspoon ground cinnamon
- Pinch of salt

Instructions:

1. Preheat your oven to 325°F (160°C). Line a baking dish or tray with parchment paper.
2. In a large bowl, combine the shredded coconut, pumpkin seeds, chopped dried apricots, and chopped dates.
3. In a small bowl, whisk together the melted coconut oil, honey or maple syrup (if using), ground cinnamon, and a pinch of salt.
4. Pour the wet mixture over the dry ingredients and stir until well combined.
5. Transfer the mixture into the lined baking dish or tray. Use a spatula or your hands to press the mixture firmly and evenly into the dish.
6. Bake in the preheated oven for 20-25 minutes, or until the edges are golden brown.
7. Allow the granola bars to cool completely in the baking dish before cutting into bars.
8. Once cooled, cut into 10 bars.
9. Serve immediately, or store in an airtight container for up to one week.

Nutritional Information per Serving:

- **Calories:** 220 kcal
- **Fat:** 15g
- **Carbohydrates:** 18g
- **Proteins:** 4g

Baked Kale Chips with Sea Salt and Olive Oil

Prep Time: 10 minutes | **Cook Time:** 15 minutes | **Servings:** 4

Ingredients:

- 1 bunch kale, washed and dried

- 2 tablespoons olive oil

- Sea salt, to taste

Instructions:

1. Preheat your oven to 300°F (150°C). Take out the tough stems from the kale leaves and tear the leaves into bite-sized pieces.

2. In a large bowl, drizzle the kale pieces with olive oil. Use your hands to massage the oil into the kale leaves until evenly coated.

3. Spread the kale pieces in a single layer on a baking sheet lined with parchment paper. Sprinkle with sea salt to taste.

4. Bake in the preheated oven for 10-15 minutes, or until the edges are crisp and slightly browned. Watch carefully to prevent burning.

5. Remove from the oven and let the kale chips cool on the baking sheet for a few minutes. Transfer to a serving bowl and enjoy immediately.

Nutritional Information per Serving:

- **Calories:** 90 kcal

- **Fat:** 7g

- **Carbohydrates:** 6g

- **Proteins:** 3g

Coconut Macaroons with Dark Chocolate Drizzle

Prep Time: 15 minutes | **Cook Time:** 20 minutes | **Servings:** 12 macaroons

Ingredients:

- 2 cups shredded coconut
- 1/2 cup coconut cream (from full-fat coconut milk)
- 1/4 cup honey or maple syrup (avoid for strict AIP)
- 1 teaspoon vanilla extract
- Pinch of salt
- 1/2 cup dark chocolate chips (ensure AIP compliant)

Instructions:

1. Preheat your oven to 325°F (160°C). Line a baking sheet with parchment paper.
2. In a mixing bowl, combine the shredded coconut, coconut cream, honey or maple syrup (if using), vanilla extract, and a pinch of salt. Mix until well combined.
3. Scoop tablespoon-sized portions of the mixture and shape them into macaroons using your hands. Place them on the prepared baking sheet.
4. Bake in the preheated oven for 18-20 minutes, or until the macaroons are lightly golden brown on the edges.
5. Remove from the oven and let the macaroons cool completely on a wire rack.
6. Melt the dark chocolate chips in a microwave-safe bowl in 30-second intervals, stirring in between, until smooth.
7. Drizzle the melted chocolate over the cooled macaroons.
8. Allow the chocolate to set at room temperature. Serve and enjoy!

Nutritional Information per Serving:

- **Calories:** 160 kcal
- **Fat:** 12g
- **Carbohydrates:** 12g
- **Proteins:** 2g

Deviled Eggs with Avocado and Smoked Paprika

Prep Time: 20 minutes | **Cook Time:** 10 minutes | **Servings:** 6

Ingredients:

- 6 large eggs
- 1 ripe avocado
- 2 tablespoons olive oil
- 1 tablespoon lemon juice
- 1/2 teaspoon smoked paprika
- Salt and pepper, to taste
- Fresh parsley or chives, chopped (for garnish)

Instructions:

1. Place the eggs in a saucepan and cover with water. Bring to a boil over medium-high heat. Once boiling, cover the pan and remove from heat. Let the eggs sit in the hot water for 10 minutes. Then, transfer the eggs to a bowl of ice water to cool.

2. Peel the cooled eggs, then slice them in half lengthwise. Carefully take out the yolks and place them in a bowl.

3. Cut the avocado in half, take out the pit, and scoop the flesh into the bowl with the egg yolks. Add olive oil, lemon juice, smoked paprika, salt, and pepper to the bowl.

4. Mash everything together with a fork until smooth and creamy. Adjust seasoning to taste.

5. Spoon or pipe the avocado mixture into the hollowed-out egg whites.

6. Sprinkle with chopped fresh parsley or chives and a pinch of smoked paprika for garnish. Serve chilled.

Nutritional Information per Serving:

- **Calories:** 140 kcal
- **Fat:** 10g
- **Carbohydrates:** 4g
- **Proteins:** 7g

Mixed Berry Fruit Leather with Honey

Prep Time: 15 minutes | **Cook Time:** 4-6 hours (drying time) | **Servings:** 6

Ingredients:

- 2 cups mixed berries (such as strawberries, blueberries, raspberries)
- 2 tablespoons honey (avoid for strict AIP)

Instructions:

1. Wash the berries thoroughly and remove any stems or leaves.

2. In a blender or food processor, combine the mixed berries and honey. Blend until smooth.

3. Pour the blended mixture into a saucepan. Cook over medium heat, stirring constantly, until the mixture thickens slightly, about 5-7 minutes.

4. Preheat your oven to the lowest setting (usually around 140-170°F or 60-75°C). Line a baking sheet with parchment paper.

5. Pour the cooked berry mixture onto the prepared baking sheet. Use a spatula to spread it evenly into a thin layer, about 1/8 inch thick.

6. Place the baking sheet in the oven and leave the door slightly ajar to allow moisture to escape. Let it dry for 4-6 hours, or until the fruit leather is dry to the touch and peels away easily from the parchment paper.

7. Remove from the oven and let it cool completely. Once cooled, cut the fruit leather into strips using kitchen shears or a sharp knife.

8. Roll each strip of fruit leather and store in an airtight container at room temperature.

Nutritional Information per Serving:

- **Calories:** 80 kcal
- **Fat:** 0.5g
- **Carbohydrates:** 20g
- **Proteins:** 1g

Plantain Chips with Guacamole and Salsa

Prep Time: 15 minutes | **Cook Time:** 15 minutes | **Servings:** 4

Ingredients:

- 2 large green plantains
- 2 tablespoons olive oil
- **Guacamole:**
  - 2 ripe avocados
  - 1 tablespoon lime juice
- **Salsa:**
  - 1 cup diced tomatoes
  - 1/4 cup diced red onion
  - 1/4 cup chopped fresh cilantro
- Salt, to taste
  - 1/4 teaspoon garlic powder
  - Salt and pepper, to taste
  - 1 tablespoon lime juice
  - Salt and pepper, to taste

Instructions:

1. Preheat your oven to 400°F (200°C). Peel the plantains and slice them thinly using a mandoline slicer or a sharp knife.

2. In a bowl, toss the plantain slices with olive oil and salt until evenly coated.

3. Arrange the plantain slices in a single layer on a baking sheet lined with parchment paper. Bake for 10-15 minutes, flipping halfway through, until the chips are golden brown and crisp.

4. In a bowl, mash the avocados with lime juice, garlic powder, salt, and pepper until smooth. Adjust seasoning to taste.

5. In another bowl, combine diced tomatoes, diced red onion, chopped cilantro, lime juice, salt, and pepper. Mix adequately.

6. Arrange the plantain chips on a serving platter. Serve with guacamole and salsa on the side.

Nutritional Information per Serving:

- **Calories:** 250 kcal
- **Fat:** 15g
- **Carbohydrates:** 30g
- **Proteins:** 2g

AIP Beef Jerky with Herbs and Garlic

Prep Time: 20 minutes | **Cook Time:** 4-6 hours (drying time) | **Servings:** 6

Ingredients:

- 1-pound lean beef, thinly sliced against the grain
- 1/4 cup coconut aminos
- 2 tablespoons apple cider vinegar
- 2 cloves garlic, minced

- 1 teaspoon dried thyme
- 1 teaspoon dried rosemary
- 1/2 teaspoon onion powder
- 1/2 teaspoon garlic powder
- Salt and pepper, to taste

Instructions:

1. Trim any visible fat from the beef and slice it thinly against the grain. This helps to ensure the jerky is tender.

2. In a bowl, combine coconut aminos, apple cider vinegar, minced garlic, dried thyme, dried rosemary, onion powder, garlic powder, salt, and pepper. Mix adequately.

3. Place the beef slices into the marinade, making sure each slice is coated evenly. Cover and refrigerate for at least 1 hour, or overnight for deeper flavor.

4. Preheat your oven to the lowest setting (usually around 140-170°F or 60-75°C). Line a baking sheet with parchment paper.

5. Take out the beef slices from the marinade and pat them dry with paper towels. Arrange the slices in a single layer on the prepared baking sheet.

6. Place the baking sheet in the oven and leave the door slightly ajar to allow moisture to escape. Dry the beef for 4-6 hours, or until the jerky is dry to the touch and bends without breaking.

7. Once dried, let the beef jerky cool completely on a wire rack. Store in an airtight container at room temperature for up to 2 weeks.

Nutritional Information per Serving:

- **Calories:** 180 kcal
- **Fat:** 6g
- **Carbohydrates:** 4g
- **Proteins:** 25g

<u>Chia Seed Pudding with Coconut Milk, Honey, and Blueberries</u>

Prep Time: 5 minutes | **Cook Time:** 0 minutes (plus chilling time) | **Servings:** 2

Ingredients:

- 1/4 cup chia seeds

- 1 cup coconut milk (full-fat)

- 1 tablespoon honey (avoid for strict AIP)

- 1/2 cup fresh blueberries

- Optional: Shredded coconut and mint leaves for garnish

Instructions:

1. In a bowl or jar, combine the chia seeds and coconut milk. Stir adequately to combine.

2. Stir in the honey, if using, until evenly distributed.

3. Cover the bowl or jar and refrigerate for at least 2 hours, or overnight, until the chia seeds have absorbed the liquid and the mixture has thickened to a pudding-like consistency.

4. Divide the chia seed pudding into serving bowls or glasses.

5. Top each serving with fresh blueberries.

6. Sprinkle with shredded coconut and garnish with mint leaves, if desired.

7. Serve chilled and enjoy!

Nutritional Information per Serving:

- **Calories:** 250 kcal

- **Fat:** 18g

- **Carbohydrates:** 18g

- **Proteins:** 5g

Sliced Cucumbers with Smoked Salmon and Dill

Prep Time: 10 minutes | **Cook Time:** 0 minutes | **Servings:** 2

Ingredients:

- 1 large cucumber, thinly sliced

- 4 ounces smoked salmon

- Fresh dill, for garnish

- Lemon wedges, for serving

Instructions:

1. Wash the cucumber thoroughly. Slice it thinly using a sharp knife or a mandoline slicer.

2. Arrange the cucumber slices on a serving platter or individual plates.

3. Place slices of smoked salmon on top of each cucumber slice.

4. Garnish with fresh dill and serve with lemon wedges on the side.

Nutritional Information per Serving:

- **Calories:** 150 kcal

- **Fat:** 7g

- **Carbohydrates:** 4g

- **Proteins:** 20g

Trail Mix with Nuts, Seeds, and Dried Fruit

Prep Time: 10 minutes | **Cook Time:** 0 minutes | **Servings:** 6

Ingredients:

- 1 cup raw almonds
- 1 cup raw cashews
- 1/2 cup pumpkin seeds
- 1/2 cup sunflower seeds
- 1/2 cup dried cranberries
- 1/2 cup dried apricots, diced
- 1/4 cup unsweetened coconut flakes

Instructions:

1. If necessary, chop the dried apricots into small pieces.

2. In a large bowl, combine the raw almonds, raw cashews, pumpkin seeds, sunflower seeds, dried cranberries, diced dried apricots, and unsweetened coconut flakes.

3. Stir the ingredients until evenly distributed.

4. Transfer the trail mix to an airtight container for storage.

5. Serve immediately, or portion out into individual servings for convenient snacking.

Nutritional Information per Serving:

- **Calories:** 280 kcal
- **Fat:** 18g
- **Carbohydrates:** 24g
- **Proteins:** 8g

Chapter 7: Reintroduction Phase

Breakfast Recipes

Spinach and Egg Yolk Salad with Lemon Dressing (Stage 1: Egg Yolks)

Prep Time: 10 minutes | **Cook Time:** 10 minutes | **Servings:** 4

Ingredients

- 6 cups fresh spinach leaves, washed and dried
- 4 large egg yolks
- 1 medium avocado, diced
- 1 tablespoon extra-virgin olive oil
- 1 tablespoon freshly squeezed lemon juice
- 1 teaspoon Dijon mustard (optional, for taste reintroduction)
- Sea salt, to taste
- Freshly ground black pepper, to taste (optional, for taste reintroduction)

Instructions

1. Place the egg yolks in a pot and cover them with water. Bring to a boil, then reduce heat and simmer for 10 minutes.
2. Take out the yolks from the water and let them cool. Once cooled, crumble the egg yolks into small pieces.
3. In a small bowl, whisk together the extra-virgin olive oil, freshly squeezed lemon juice, and Dijon mustard (if using).
4. Season with sea salt and freshly ground black pepper (if using) to taste.
5. In a large salad bowl, add the fresh spinach leaves and diced avocado.
6. Add the crumbled egg yolks on top of the spinach and avocado.
7. Drizzle the lemon dressing over the salad and gently toss to combine.
8. Divide the salad evenly among four plates and serve immediately.

Nutritional Information (per serving)

- **Calories:** 180 kcal
- **Fat:** 15 g
- **Carbohydrates:** 6 g
- **Protein:** 6 g

Banana Pancakes with Almond Butter (Stage 2: Almonds)

Prep Time: 10 minutes | **Cook Time:** 10 minutes | **Servings:** 2

Ingredients

- 2 large ripe bananas, mashed
- 2 large egg yolks
- 1 teaspoon vanilla extract
- 1 teaspoon ground cinnamon
- 1 tablespoon coconut flour
- 1 tablespoon almond butter
- 1 teaspoon coconut oil (for cooking)

Instructions

1. In a mixing bowl, combine the mashed bananas, large egg yolks, vanilla extract, and ground cinnamon.

2. Add the coconut flour to the banana mixture and mix until well combined.

3. Heat the coconut oil in a large non-stick skillet over medium heat.

4. Pour small portions of the batter into the skillet to form pancakes.

5. Cook each pancake for about 2-3 minutes on each side, or until golden brown and cooked through.

6. Place the cooked pancakes on a plate.

7. Spread almond butter on top of each pancake.

8. You may add additional slices of banana or a drizzle of honey (if tolerated) as toppings.

Nutritional Information (per serving)

- **Calories:** 250 kcal
- **Fat:** 15 g
- **Carbohydrates:** 26 g
- **Protein:** 6 g

<u>Sweet Potato Hash with Cashew Cream (Stage 2: Cashews)</u>

Prep Time: 15 minutes | **Cook Time:** 20 minutes | **Servings:** 4

Ingredients

- 2 large sweet potatoes, peeled and diced
- 1 medium onion, diced
- 1 red bell pepper, diced
- 2 tablespoons extra-virgin olive oil
- 1 teaspoon sea salt
- 1 teaspoon garlic powder
- 1 teaspoon dried thyme
- 1/2 cup raw cashews (soaked in water for at least 2 hours)
- 1/4 cup water
- 1 tablespoon lemon juice
- Sea salt, to taste (for the cashew cream)
- Freshly ground black pepper, to taste (optional, for taste reintroduction)

Instructions

1. Drain the soaked raw cashews and place them in a blender.
2. Add the water, lemon juice, sea salt, and freshly ground black pepper (if using).
3. Blend until smooth and creamy. Adjust the seasoning to taste.
4. Heat the extra-virgin olive oil in a large skillet over medium heat.
5. Add the diced onion and diced red bell pepper, and sauté for about 5 minutes, until softened.
6. Add the diced sweet potatoes, sea salt, garlic powder, and dried thyme. Stir to combine.
7. Cover the skillet and cook for about 15 minutes, stirring occasionally, until the sweet potatoes are tender and slightly crispy.
8. Divide the sweet potato hash evenly among four plates.
9. Drizzle the cashew cream over the top of each serving.

Nutritional Information (per serving)

- **Calories:** 300 kcal
- **Fat:** 18 g
- **Carbohydrates:** 30 g
- **Protein:** 6 g

Chia Seed Pudding with Berries (Stage 2: Chia Seeds)

Prep Time: 10 minutes | **Cook Time:** 0 minutes (plus 4 hours of chilling) | **Servings:** 4

Ingredients

- 1/2 cup chia seeds
- 2 cups unsweetened almond milk
- 1 teaspoon vanilla extract
- 1 tablespoon maple syrup (optional, for taste reintroduction)
- 1 cup mixed berries (fresh or frozen)

Instructions

1. In a medium bowl, combine the chia seeds, unsweetened almond milk, vanilla extract, and maple syrup (if using).
2. Stir adequately to ensure the chia seeds are evenly distributed.
3. Cover the bowl and refrigerate for at least 4 hours or overnight, until the mixture has thickened to a pudding-like consistency.
4. Divide the chia seed pudding evenly among four serving bowls.
5. Top each serving with mixed berries.

Nutritional Information (per serving)

- **Calories:** 160 kcal
- **Fat:** 8 g
- **Carbohydrates:** 18 g
- **Protein:** 4 g

Scrambled Eggs with Avocado and Salsa (Stage 1: Whole Eggs)

Prep Time: 10 minutes | **Cook Time:** 5 minutes | **Servings:** 2

Ingredients

- 4 large eggs, whisked
- 1 tablespoon extra-virgin olive oil
- 1 medium avocado, diced
- 1/2 cup fresh salsa (store-bought or homemade)
- Sea salt, to taste
- Freshly ground black pepper, to taste (optional, for taste reintroduction)

Instructions

1. Heat the extra-virgin olive oil in a non-stick skillet over medium heat.
2. Pour the whisked eggs into the skillet and cook, stirring gently, until the eggs are scrambled and cooked through. Season with sea salt and freshly ground black pepper (if using) to taste.
3. Divide the scrambled eggs evenly between two plates.
4. Top each serving with the diced avocado and fresh salsa.

Nutritional Information (per serving)

- **Calories:** 280 kcal
- **Fat:** 22 g
- **Carbohydrates:** 10 g
- **Protein:** 14 g

Breakfast Smoothie with Flax Seeds (Stage 2: Flax Seeds)

Prep Time: 5 minutes | **Cook Time:** 0 minutes | **Servings:** 2

Ingredients

- 1 cup unsweetened almond milk
- 1 medium banana, sliced
- 1/2 cup fresh or frozen berries (e.g., blueberries, strawberries)
- 1 tablespoon ground flax seeds
- 1 tablespoon almond butter
- 1 teaspoon vanilla extract
- 1 handful spinach leaves, washed and dried

Instructions

1. In a blender, combine the unsweetened almond milk, sliced banana, fresh or frozen berries, ground flax seeds, almond butter, vanilla extract, and spinach leaves.

2. Blend until smooth and creamy.

3. Pour the smoothie into two glasses and serve immediately.

Nutritional Information (per serving)

- **Calories:** 220 kcal
- **Fat:** 10 g
- **Carbohydrates:** 26 g
- **Protein:** 6 g

Egg Muffins with Spinach and Mushrooms (Stage 1: Whole Eggs)

Prep Time: 10 minutes | **Cook Time:** 20 minutes | **Servings:** 4

Ingredients

- 8 large eggs, whisked
- 1 cup fresh spinach leaves, chopped
- 1 cup mushrooms, diced
- 1/4 cup unsweetened almond milk
- 1 tablespoon extra-virgin olive oil
- Sea salt, to taste
- Freshly ground black pepper, to taste (optional, for taste reintroduction)

Instructions

1. Preheat the oven to 350 degrees Fahrenheit (175 degrees Celsius).
2. Grease a 12-cup muffin tin with extra-virgin olive oil.
3. Heat the extra-virgin olive oil in a skillet over medium heat.
4. Add the diced mushrooms and cook for about 5 minutes until softened.
5. Add the chopped spinach leaves and cook for another 2 minutes until wilted. Remove from heat.
6. In a large bowl, combine the whisked eggs, unsweetened almond milk, sea salt, and freshly ground black pepper (if using).
7. Stir in the cooked mushrooms and spinach.
8. Pour the egg mixture evenly into the greased muffin tin cups.
9. Bake in the preheated oven for about 15-20 minutes, or until the eggs are set and a toothpick inserted into the center comes out clean.
10. Allow the egg muffins to cool slightly before removing them from the tin.
11. Serve warm.

Nutritional Information (per serving)

- **Calories:** 160 kcal
- **Fat:** 11 g
- **Carbohydrates:** 3 g
- **Protein:** 12 g

Butternut Squash Breakfast Bowl with Pumpkin Seeds (Stage 2: Pumpkin Seeds)

Prep Time: 10 minutes | **Cook Time:** 20 minutes | **Servings:** 2

Ingredients

- 2 cups butternut squash, peeled and diced
- 1 tablespoon extra-virgin olive oil
- 1/4 teaspoon sea salt
- 1/4 teaspoon ground cinnamon
- 2 tablespoons pumpkin seeds
- 1 tablespoon unsweetened shredded coconut (optional)
- 1/2 cup unsweetened almond milk
- 1 teaspoon maple syrup (optional, for taste reintroduction)

Instructions

1. Preheat the oven to 400 degrees Fahrenheit (200 degrees Celsius).

2. Place the diced butternut squash on a baking sheet and drizzle with extra-virgin olive oil. Sprinkle with sea salt and ground cinnamon.

3. Roast in the preheated oven for about 20 minutes, or until the squash is tender and slightly caramelized.

4. In a small dry skillet over medium heat, toast the pumpkin seeds for 2-3 minutes, stirring frequently, until they are golden brown and fragrant.

5. Divide the roasted butternut squash evenly between two bowls.

6. Top each bowl with toasted pumpkin seeds and unsweetened shredded coconut (if using).

7. Drizzle with unsweetened almond milk and maple syrup (if using).

Nutritional Information (per serving)

- **Calories:** 200 kcal
- **Fat:** 12 g
- **Carbohydrates:** 20 g
- **Protein:** 4 g

Avocado Toast on AIP Bread with Egg Yolk (Stage 1: Egg Yolks)

Prep Time: 10 minutes | **Cook Time:** 10 minutes | **Servings:** 2

Ingredients

- 2 slices AIP bread (such as cassava or coconut flour bread)
- 1 ripe avocado
- 2 large egg yolks
- 1 tablespoon extra-virgin olive oil
- Sea salt, to taste
- Freshly ground black pepper, to taste (optional, for taste reintroduction)

Instructions

1. Toast the AIP bread slices until golden brown and crispy.
2. Cut the ripe avocado in half, take out the pit, and scoop the flesh into a small bowl.
3. Mash the avocado with a fork until smooth. Season with sea salt to taste.
4. Heat the extra-virgin olive oil in a non-stick skillet over medium heat.
5. Carefully crack each egg and separate the yolks. Place the egg yolks in the skillet.
6. Cook the egg yolks gently for about 2-3 minutes, until the whites are set but the yolks are still runny.
7. Spread the mashed avocado evenly onto each slice of toasted AIP bread.
8. Carefully place one cooked egg yolk on top of each avocado toast.
9. Season with freshly ground black pepper (if using) to taste.
10. Serve the avocado toast immediately while warm.

Nutritional Information (per serving)

- **Calories:** 300 kcal
- **Fat:** 20 g
- **Carbohydrates:** 20 g
- **Protein:** 10 g

Mixed Berry Smoothie with Hemp Seeds (Stage 2: Hemp Seeds)

Prep Time: 5 minutes | **Cook Time:** 0 minutes | **Servings:** 2

Ingredients

- 1 cup mixed berries (fresh or frozen)
- 1 cup unsweetened almond milk
- 2 tablespoons hemp seeds
- 1 tablespoon almond butter
- 1 teaspoon vanilla extract

Instructions

1. In a blender, combine the mixed berries, unsweetened almond milk, hemp seeds, almond butter, and vanilla extract.
2. Blend until smooth and creamy.
3. Pour the smoothie into two glasses.

Nutritional Information (per serving)

- **Calories:** 180 kcal
- **Fat:** 10 g
- **Carbohydrates:** 15 g
- **Protein:** 7 g

AIP Breakfast Sausage with Poached Eggs (Stage 1: Whole Eggs)

Prep Time: 15 minutes | **Cook Time:** 15 minutes | **Servings:** 2

Ingredients

AIP Breakfast Sausage:

- 1/2-pound ground pork
- 1/2 teaspoon dried sage
- 1/2 teaspoon dried thyme
- 1/2 teaspoon garlic powder
- 1/4 teaspoon sea salt
- 1/4 teaspoon ground black pepper (omit for AIP)

Poached Eggs:

- 4 large eggs
- Water, for poaching
- 1 tablespoon white vinegar (optional, for poaching)

Instructions

1. In a bowl, combine the ground pork, dried sage, dried thyme, garlic powder, sea salt, and ground black pepper (if using).
2. Mix adequately until the spices are evenly distributed.
3. Form the mixture into small patties, about 2 inches in diameter.
4. Heat a skillet over medium heat.
5. Add the sausage patties to the skillet and cook for about 4-5 minutes on each side, or until fully cooked through and browned. Remove from heat and set aside.
6. Fill a medium saucepan with water and bring to a simmer.
7. Add the white vinegar (if using) to the simmering water.
8. Crack each egg into a small bowl or ramekin.
9. Gently slide each egg into the simmering water, one at a time.
10. Cook the eggs for about 3-4 minutes, until the whites are set but the yolks are still runny.
11. Place two sausage patties on each serving plate.
12. Carefully take out the poached eggs from the water using a slotted spoon and place one egg on top of each sausage patty.
13. Season with additional sea salt and ground black pepper if desired.
14. Serve the AIP breakfast sausage with poached eggs immediately while warm.

Nutritional Information (per serving)

- **Calories:** 320 kcal
- **Fat:** 24 g
- **Carbohydrates:** 1 g
- **Protein:** 26 g

Lunch Recipes

Grilled Chicken Salad with Sesame Dressing (Stage 2: Sesame Seeds)

Prep Time: 15 minutes | **Cook Time:** 15 minutes | **Number of Servings:** 4

Ingredients:

- 500g boneless, skinless chicken breasts
- 1 tbsp olive oil
- Salt and pepper, to taste
- 4 cups mixed salad greens (e.g., spinach, arugula)
- 1 large cucumber, sliced
- 1 medium carrot, shredded
- 1/4 cup sliced red onion
- 2 tbsp sesame seeds, toasted
- Fresh cilantro or parsley for garnish

Sesame Dressing:

- 3 tbsp olive oil
- 2 tbsp apple cider vinegar
- 1 tbsp coconut aminos
- 1 tbsp sesame oil
- 1 tsp honey (optional, omit for stricter AIP)
- Salt and pepper, to taste

Instructions:

1. Preheat grill to medium-high heat.
2. Season chicken breasts with olive oil, salt, and pepper.
3. Grill chicken breasts for about 6-7 minutes per side or until fully cooked (internal temperature of 165°F or 74°C). Remove from grill and let rest for 5 minutes before slicing.
4. In a large bowl, combine mixed greens, sliced cucumber, shredded carrot, and sliced red onion.
5. In a small bowl, whisk together olive oil, apple cider vinegar, coconut aminos, sesame oil, honey (if using), salt, and pepper.
6. Divide the salad mixture onto serving plates. Top each salad with sliced grilled chicken.
7. Drizzle with sesame dressing and sprinkle toasted sesame seeds over each salad.
8. Garnish with fresh cilantro or parsley.

Nutritional Information (per serving):

- **Calories:** 320 kcal
- **Fat:** 18g
- **Carbohydrates:** 10g
- **Proteins:** 28g

Turkey Wraps with Almond Flour Tortillas (Stage 2: Almond Flour)

Prep Time: 20 minutes | **Cook Time:** 10 minutes | **Number of Servings:** 4

Ingredients:

- 500g ground turkey
- 1 tbsp olive oil
- Salt and pepper, to taste
- 1/2 tsp garlic powder
- 1/2 tsp onion powder
- 1/2 tsp dried oregano

- 4 almond flour tortillas (store-bought or homemade)
- 1 cup shredded lettuce
- 1 medium tomato, diced
- 1/2 avocado, sliced
- 1/4 cup sliced black olives
- Fresh cilantro for garnish

Instructions:

1. In a skillet, heat olive oil over medium heat.
2. Season ground turkey with salt, pepper, garlic powder, onion powder, and dried oregano. Cook in the skillet until browned and fully cooked, breaking it apart with a spoon as it cooks, about 8-10 minutes.
3. Warm almond flour tortillas according to package instructions or preference.
4. Divide cooked turkey equally among the tortillas.
5. Top each tortilla with shredded lettuce, diced tomato, avocado slices, and sliced black olives.
6. Fold the sides of each tortilla towards the center, then roll up tightly to enclose the filling.
7. Slice each wrap in half diagonally.
8. Arrange on a serving plate, garnish with fresh cilantro if desired, and serve immediately.

Nutritional Information (per serving):

- **Calories:** 380 kcal
- **Fat:** 22g
- **Carbohydrates:** 19g
- **Proteins:** 28g

Mixed Greens Salad with Egg Yolk Vinaigrette (Stage 1: Egg Yolks)

Prep Time: 15 minutes | **Cook Time:** 10 minutes | **Number of Servings:** 4

Ingredients:

- 4 large egg yolks, boiled and peeled
- 1/4 cup olive oil
- 2 tbsp apple cider vinegar
- 1 tbsp lemon juice
- 1 tsp Dijon mustard
- Salt and pepper, to taste

- 6 cups mixed salad greens (e.g., spinach, arugula, romaine)
- 1/2 cucumber, sliced
- 1/4 red onion, thinly sliced
- 1/4 cup cherry tomatoes, halved
- 1/4 cup sliced avocado

Instructions:

1. In a small bowl, mash the boiled egg yolks with a fork until smooth.
2. Whisk in olive oil, apple cider vinegar, lemon juice, Dijon mustard, salt, and pepper until well combined. Set aside.
3. In a large bowl, combine mixed salad greens, cucumber slices, red onion, cherry tomatoes, and avocado slices.
4. Drizzle the egg yolk vinaigrette over the salad and toss gently to coat evenly.
5. Divide the salad into four bowls and serve immediately.

Nutritional Information (per serving):

- **Calories:** 280 kcal
- **Fat:** 20g
- **Carbohydrates:** 8g
- **Proteins:** 12g

<u>Beef Stir-fry with Bell Peppers (Stage 3: Bell Peppers)</u>

Prep Time: 15 minutes | **Cook Time:** 15 minutes | **Number of Servings:** 4

Ingredients:

- 500g beef sirloin, thinly sliced
- 2 tbsp coconut aminos
- 1 tbsp olive oil
- 1/2 tsp garlic powder
- 1/2 tsp onion powder
- 1/2 tsp ground ginger
- Salt and pepper, to taste
- 2 bell peppers (any color), sliced
- 1 medium zucchini, sliced
- 1 cup broccoli florets
- Fresh cilantro for garnish

Instructions:

1. In a bowl, combine sliced beef sirloin with coconut aminos, garlic powder, onion powder, ground ginger, salt, and pepper. Let it marinate for at least 10 minutes.

2. Heat olive oil in a large skillet or wok over medium-high heat.

3. Add the marinated beef and stir-fry for 3-4 minutes until browned and cooked through. Remove from skillet and set aside.

4. In the same skillet, add bell peppers, zucchini, and broccoli florets. Stir-fry for 5-6 minutes until vegetables are tender-crisp.

5. Return the cooked beef to the skillet with the vegetables. Stir everything together and cook for another 1-2 minutes to heat through.

6. Divide the beef stir-fry among serving plates.

7. Garnish with fresh cilantro before serving.

Nutritional Information (per serving):

- **Calories:** 340 kcal
- **Fat:** 15g
- **Carbohydrates:** 12g
- **Proteins:** 35g

Salmon Salad with Avocado and Flaxseed Oil (Stage 2: Flaxseed Oil)

Prep Time: 15 minutes | **Cook Time:** 15 minutes (for salmon, if not using pre-cooked) | **Number of Servings:** 4

Ingredients:

- 500g salmon fillets, cooked and flaked (or canned salmon)
- 1 avocado, diced
- 1/4 cup cucumber, diced
- 1/4 cup red bell pepper, diced
- 2 tbsp red onion, finely chopped
- 2 tbsp fresh dill, chopped
- 2 tbsp flaxseed oil
- Juice of 1 lemon
- Salt and pepper, to taste
- Mixed salad greens for serving

Instructions:

1. If using fresh salmon, preheat the oven to 375°F (190°C). Season salmon fillets with salt and pepper, bake for 12-15 minutes until cooked through, then flake into pieces. Let it cool.

2. In a large bowl, combine flaked salmon, diced avocado, cucumber, red bell pepper, red onion, and fresh dill.

3. In a small bowl, whisk together flaxseed oil, lemon juice, salt, and pepper.

4. Pour the dressing over the salmon and vegetable mixture. Toss gently to combine.

5. Serve the salmon salad over a bed of mixed salad greens.

Nutritional Information (per serving):

- **Calories:** 320 kcal
- **Fat:** 20g
- **Carbohydrates:** 8g
- **Proteins:** 28g

Zucchini Noodles with Walnut Pesto (Stage 2: Walnuts)

Prep Time: 20 minutes | **Cook Time:** 10 minutes | **Number of Servings:** 4

Ingredients:

- 4 medium zucchinis, spiralized into noodles
- 1 cup fresh basil leaves
- 1/2 cup walnuts
- 1/4 cup olive oil
- 2 cloves garlic, minced
- Juice of 1 lemon
- Salt and pepper, to taste
- Cherry tomatoes, halved, for garnish (optional)
- Fresh basil leaves, chopped, for garnish (optional)

Instructions:

1. In a food processor, combine basil leaves, walnuts, olive oil, minced garlic, lemon juice, salt, and pepper. Blend until smooth and creamy. Set aside.

2. Heat a large skillet over medium heat. Add zucchini noodles and sauté for 3-4 minutes until just tender. Drain excess liquid if necessary.

3. Add the walnut pesto to the skillet with the zucchini noodles. Toss gently to coat the noodles evenly with the pesto sauce.

4. Divide the zucchini noodles with walnut pesto among serving plates.

5. Garnish with halved cherry tomatoes and chopped fresh basil leaves if desired.

Nutritional Information (per serving):

- **Calories:** 280 kcal
- **Fat:** 22g
- **Carbohydrates:** 12g
- **Proteins:** 8g

Chicken Caesar Salad with Egg Yolks in Dressing (Stage 1: Egg Yolks)

Prep Time: 20 minutes | **Cook Time:** 15 minutes | **Number of Servings:** 4

Ingredients:

- 500g chicken breasts, grilled and sliced
- 1 head romaine lettuce, chopped
- 1/2 cup cherry tomatoes, halved
- 1/4 cup sliced red onion
- 1/4 cup grated Parmesan cheese (optional, omit for stricter AIP)
- Fresh parsley for garnish

Egg Yolk Dressing:

- 4 large egg yolks, hard-boiled and peeled
- 1/4 cup olive oil
- 2 tbsp lemon juice
- 1 clove garlic, minced
- 1 tsp Dijon mustard
- Salt and pepper, to taste

Instructions:

1. Grill chicken breasts until cooked through, about 6-7 minutes per side. Let them rest for 5 minutes before slicing.

2. In a bowl, mash the hard-boiled egg yolks with a fork until smooth.

3. Whisk in olive oil, lemon juice, minced garlic, Dijon mustard, salt, and pepper until well combined. Adjust seasoning to taste.

4. In a large bowl, combine chopped romaine lettuce, cherry tomatoes, sliced red onion, and grated Parmesan cheese (if using).

5. Pour the egg yolk dressing over the salad mixture. Toss gently to coat everything evenly with the dressing.

6. Arrange sliced grilled chicken on top of the dressed salad.

7. Garnish with fresh parsley before serving.

Nutritional Information (per serving):

- **Calories:** 340 kcal
- **Fat:** 20g
- **Carbohydrates:** 6g
- **Proteins:** 32g

AIP BLT Salad with Avocado and Tomato (Stage 3: Tomatoes)

Prep Time: 15 minutes | **Cook Time:** 10 minutes | **Number of Servings:** 4

Ingredients:

- 500g bacon, cooked until crispy and chopped
- 2 avocados, diced
- 2 large tomatoes, diced
- 1/4 cup red onion, thinly sliced
- 6 cups mixed salad greens (e.g., spinach, arugula, romaine)
- Fresh parsley for garnish

Instructions:

1. Cook bacon until crispy, then chop into pieces.
2. Dice avocados and tomatoes. Thinly slice red onion.
3. In a large bowl, combine mixed salad greens, diced avocados, diced tomatoes, sliced red onion, and chopped crispy bacon.
4. Toss the salad gently to mix all ingredients evenly.
5. Divide the salad among serving plates.
6. Garnish with fresh parsley before serving.

Nutritional Information (per serving):

- **Calories:** 420 kcal
- **Fat:** 30g
- **Carbohydrates:** 12g
- **Proteins:** 28g

Shrimp and Mango Salad with Sesame Seeds (Stage 2: Sesame Seeds)

Prep Time: 20 minutes | **Cook Time:** 5 minutes | **Number of Servings:** 4

Ingredients:

- 500g shrimp, peeled and deveined
- 2 mangos, peeled and diced
- 1/4 cup red bell pepper, diced
- 1/4 cup red onion, finely chopped
- 1/4 cup fresh cilantro, chopped
- 2 tbsp sesame seeds
- Mixed salad greens for serving

Sesame Dressing:

- 1/4 cup sesame oil
- 2 tbsp rice vinegar
- 1 tbsp coconut aminos
- 1 clove garlic, minced
- Salt and pepper, to taste

Instructions:

1. Heat a skillet over medium-high heat. Add shrimp and cook for 2-3 minutes per side until pink and cooked through. Remove from heat and set aside.

2. Dice the peeled mangoes, red bell pepper, and finely chop the red onion. Chop the fresh cilantro.

3. In a small bowl, whisk together sesame oil, rice vinegar, coconut aminos, minced garlic, salt, and pepper until well combined.

4. In a large bowl, combine mixed salad greens, cooked shrimp, diced mangoes, diced red bell pepper, chopped red onion, and fresh cilantro.

5. Drizzle the sesame dressing over the salad mixture.

6. Sprinkle sesame seeds over the salad as a final touch.

7. Divide the shrimp and mango salad among serving plates.

Nutritional Information (per serving):

- **Calories:** 320 kcal
- **Fat:** 18g
- **Carbohydrates:** 22g
- **Proteins:** 20g

Turkey and Cranberry Salad with Pecans (Stage 2: Pecans)

Prep Time: 15 minutes | **Cook Time:** 10 minutes (if cooking turkey) | **Number of Servings:** 4

Ingredients:

- 500g cooked turkey breast, diced
- 1/2 cup dried cranberries
- 1/4 cup pecans, chopped
- 1/4 cup celery, finely chopped
- 1/4 cup red onion, finely chopped
- 1/4 cup fresh parsley, chopped
- Mixed salad greens for serving

Dressing:

- 1/4 cup olive oil
- 2 tbsp apple cider vinegar
- 1 tbsp honey (optional, omit for stricter AIP)
- 1 clove garlic, minced
- Salt and pepper, to taste

Instructions:

1. If not using pre-cooked turkey, cook turkey breast until fully cooked and dice into bite-sized pieces. Let it cool.

2. In a large bowl, combine diced turkey, dried cranberries, chopped pecans, finely chopped celery, finely chopped red onion, and chopped fresh parsley.

3. In a small bowl, whisk together olive oil, apple cider vinegar, honey (if using), minced garlic, salt, and pepper until well combined.

4. Pour the dressing over the salad mixture. Toss gently to coat everything evenly with the dressing.

5. Serve the turkey and cranberry salad over a bed of mixed salad greens.

Nutritional Information (per serving):

- **Calories:** 380 kcal
- **Fat:** 22g
- **Carbohydrates:** 18g
- **Proteins:** 28g

Spinach and Mushroom Salad with Poached Eggs (Stage 1: Whole Eggs)

Prep Time: 15 minutes | **Cook Time:** 10 minutes | **Number of Servings:** 2

Ingredients:

- 4 large eggs
- 4 cups fresh spinach leaves
- 1 cup mushrooms, sliced
- 1/4 cup red onion, thinly sliced
- 1 tbsp olive oil
- Salt and pepper, to taste
- Fresh parsley for garnish

Instructions:

1. Fill a medium-sized saucepan with water and bring it to a gentle simmer over medium heat.

2. Crack each egg into a small bowl or ramekin. Carefully slide each egg into the simmering water. Poach for 3-4 minutes until the whites are set but the yolks are still runny. Remove with a slotted spoon and set aside.

3. Heat olive oil in a skillet over medium heat. Add sliced mushrooms and sauté for about 5 minutes until they are tender and browned. Season with salt and pepper to taste.

4. In a large bowl, combine fresh spinach leaves, thinly sliced red onion, and sautéed mushrooms.

5. Divide the spinach and mushroom mixture onto serving plates.

6. Carefully place poached eggs on top of each serving of spinach and mushrooms.

7. Garnish with fresh parsley before serving.

Nutritional Information (per serving):

- **Calories:** 280 kcal
- **Fat:** 18g
- **Carbohydrates:** 10g
- **Proteins:** 20g

Dinner Recipes

Tomato-Basil Chicken with a side of Roasted Sweet Potatoes (Stage 3: Tomatoes)

Prep Time: 15 minutes | **Cook Time:** 30 minutes | **Servings:** 4

Ingredients:

- 4 boneless, skinless chicken breasts (about 600g), pounded to an even thickness
- 4 medium sweet potatoes (about 800g), peeled and diced into 1-inch cubes
- 4 large tomatoes (about 600g), sliced
- 1/4 cup fresh basil leaves, chopped
- 4 cloves garlic, minced
- 2 tablespoons olive oil
- Salt and pepper, to taste

Instructions:

1. Preheat your oven to 400°F (200°C).

2. Place the diced sweet potatoes on a baking sheet. Drizzle with 1 tablespoon of olive oil, season with salt and pepper, and toss to coat evenly. Roast in the preheated oven for 25-30 minutes, or until tender and lightly browned.

3. In a large skillet, heat the remaining 1 tablespoon of olive oil over medium-high heat. Season the chicken breasts with salt and pepper. Cook the chicken for about 6-7 minutes per side, or until golden brown and cooked through (internal temperature of 165°F or 74°C). Remove from skillet and set aside.

4. In the same skillet, add the minced garlic and cook for about 1 minute, until fragrant. Add the sliced tomatoes and cook for another 3-4 minutes, until the tomatoes soften slightly. Stir in the chopped basil and season with salt and pepper to taste.

5. Place each chicken breast on a plate, spoon the tomato-basil mixture over the chicken, and serve with a portion of the roasted sweet potatoes.

Nutritional Information (per serving):

- **Calories:** 380 kcal
- **Fat:** 12 g
- **Carbohydrates:** 36 g
- **Proteins:** 32 g

<u>Grilled Steak with Chimichurri Sauce (Stage 3: Peppers)</u>

Prep Time: 15 minutes | **Cook Time:** 10 minutes | **Servings:** 4

Ingredients:

- 4 beef steaks (such as sirloin or ribeye), about 600g total
- 1 bunch fresh parsley, finely chopped (about 1 cup)
- 4 cloves garlic, minced
- 1/2 cup olive oil
- 2 tablespoons red wine vinegar
- 1 teaspoon dried oregano
- Salt and pepper, to taste
- 1 red bell pepper, diced

Instructions:

1. Prepare the chimichurri sauce: In a small bowl, combine the finely chopped parsley, minced garlic, olive oil, red wine vinegar, dried oregano, diced red bell pepper, salt, and pepper. Mix adequately and set aside to let the flavors meld.

2. Preheat your grill or grill pan to medium-high heat.

3. Season the steaks generously with salt and pepper. Grill the steaks for about 4-5 minutes per side, or until they reach your desired level of doneness. For medium-rare, aim for an internal temperature of 130-135°F (54-57°C).

4. Take out the steaks from the grill and let them rest for about 5 minutes before slicing.

5. Slice the steaks against the grain and drizzle with the chimichurri sauce. Serve with a side of steamed or roasted vegetables, if desired.

Nutritional Information (per serving):

- **Calories:** 480 kcal
- **Fat:** 35 g
- **Carbohydrates:** 3 g
- **Proteins:** 38 g

Pork Tenderloin with Apple and Walnut Stuffing (Stage 2: Walnuts)

Prep Time: 20 minutes | **Cook Time:** 30 minutes | **Servings:** 4

Ingredients:

- 1 pork tenderloin (about 600g)
- 1 apple, peeled, cored, and diced
- 1/2 cup walnuts, chopped
- 2 tablespoons fresh parsley, chopped
- 1 tablespoon olive oil
- Salt and pepper, to taste
- 1/2 cup chicken broth

Instructions:

1. Preheat your oven to 375°F (190°C).

2. In a bowl, combine the diced apple, chopped walnuts, chopped parsley, olive oil, salt, and pepper.

3. Using a sharp knife, make a lengthwise slit down the center of the tenderloin to create a pocket, being careful not to cut all the way through. Stuff the tenderloin with the apple and walnut mixture, pressing it gently into the pocket.

4. Season the outside of the tenderloin with salt and pepper.

5. Heat an oven-safe skillet over medium-high heat. Sear the stuffed pork tenderloin on all sides until browned, about 2-3 minutes per side.

6. Pour the chicken broth into the skillet around the pork tenderloin. Transfer the skillet to the preheated oven and roast for 20-25 minutes, or until the internal temperature reaches 145°F (63°C).

7. Take out the pork tenderloin from the oven and let it rest for 5-10 minutes before slicing. This allows the juices to redistribute.

8. Slice the pork tenderloin into rounds and serve with a portion of the apple and walnut stuffing. Optionally, drizzle with any pan juices from the skillet.

Nutritional Information (per serving):

- **Calories:** 320 kcal
- **Fat:** 14 g
- **Carbohydrates:** 8 g
- **Proteins:** 38 g

Lemon-Garlic Shrimp with Spaghetti Squash and Pesto (Stage 2: Pine Nuts)

Prep Time: 20 minutes | **Cook Time:** 40 minutes | **Servings:** 4

Ingredients:

- 1 large spaghetti squash (about 1.5 kg)
- 500g shrimp, peeled and deveined
- 4 cloves garlic, minced
- Zest and juice of 1 lemon
- 2 tablespoons olive oil
- Salt and pepper, to taste
- 1/2 cup pine nuts
- 1/2 cup fresh basil leaves
- 1/4 cup olive oil
- Salt and pepper, to taste

Instructions:

1. Preheat your oven to 400°F (200°C). Cut the spaghetti squash in half lengthwise and scoop out the seeds. Place the squash halves cut-side down on a baking sheet lined with parchment paper. Bake for 30-40 minutes, or until the squash is tender and the flesh shreds easily with a fork. Once cooked, use a fork to scrape the squash into "spaghetti" strands and set aside.

2. In a food processor, combine the pine nuts, fresh basil leaves, olive oil, salt, and pepper. Blend until smooth and set aside.

3. In a large skillet, heat 1 tablespoon of olive oil over medium-high heat. Add the minced garlic and cook for about 1 minute until fragrant. Add the shrimp, lemon zest, lemon juice, salt, and pepper. Cook the shrimp for 3-4 minutes, stirring occasionally, until they are pink and opaque.

4. Add the cooked spaghetti squash "noodles" to the skillet with the shrimp. Pour the pesto over the squash and shrimp mixture. Gently toss everything together until well combined and heated through.

5. Divide the lemon-garlic shrimp with spaghetti squash and pesto among plates. Optionally, garnish with additional pine nuts and fresh basil leaves.

Nutritional Information (per serving):

- **Calories:** 380 kcal
- **Fat:** 20 g
- **Carbohydrates:** 22 g
- **Proteins:** 30 g

Beef and Vegetable Skewers with Bell Peppers (Stage 3: Bell Peppers)

Prep Time: 20 minutes | **Cook Time:** 10 minutes | **Servings:** 4

Ingredients:

- 600g beef sirloin or tenderloin, cut into 1-inch cubes
- 2 bell peppers (1 red, 1 yellow), seeded and cut into chunks
- 1 red onion, cut into chunks
- 2 tablespoons olive oil
- 2 cloves garlic, minced
- 1 teaspoon dried oregano
- Salt and pepper, to taste

Instructions:

1. If using wooden skewers, soak them in water for at least 30 minutes to prevent burning. Thread the beef cubes, bell pepper chunks, and red onion onto the skewers, alternating ingredients.

2. In a small bowl, combine the olive oil, minced garlic, dried oregano, salt, and pepper. Brush the marinade over the beef and vegetables on the skewers, coating them evenly.

3. Preheat your grill or grill pan to medium-high heat.

4. Place the skewers on the preheated grill. Grill for about 3-4 minutes per side, or until the beef is cooked to your desired doneness and the vegetables are tender-crisp.

5. Take out the skewers from the grill and let them rest for a few minutes before serving. Optionally, serve with a side of cauliflower rice or a mixed green salad.

Nutritional Information (per serving):

- **Calories:** 380 kcal
- **Fat:** 22 g
- **Carbohydrates:** 8 g
- **Proteins:** 38 g

Herb-Crusted Salmon with Flaxseed Crust (Stage 2: Flax Seeds)

Prep Time: 15 minutes | **Cook Time:** 15 minutes | **Servings:** 4

Ingredients:

- 4 salmon fillets (about 150g each), skin-on
- 1/2 cup ground flax seeds
- 2 tablespoons fresh parsley, finely chopped
- 2 tablespoons fresh dill, finely chopped
- Zest of 1 lemon
- 2 tablespoons olive oil
- Salt and pepper, to taste

Instructions:

1. Preheat your oven to 400°F (200°C). Line a baking sheet with parchment paper.
2. In a shallow dish, combine the ground flax seeds, chopped parsley, chopped dill, lemon zest, salt, and pepper.
3. Pat the salmon fillets dry with paper towels. Brush each fillet with olive oil, then press the flaxseed mixture onto the flesh side of each fillet to coat evenly.
4. Place the salmon fillets skin-side down on the prepared baking sheet. Bake for 12-15 minutes, or until the salmon is cooked through and flakes easily with a fork.
5. Take out the salmon from the oven and let it rest for a few minutes before serving. Serve with a side of steamed vegetables or a mixed green salad.

Nutritional Information (per serving):

- **Calories:** 320 kcal
- **Fat:** 20 g
- **Carbohydrates:** 3 g
- **Proteins:** 32 g

Chicken Alfredo with Cashew Cream Sauce (Stage 2: Cashews)

Prep Time: 20 minutes | **Cook Time:** 20 minutes | **Servings:** 4

Ingredients:

- 400g boneless, skinless chicken breasts, cut into thin strips
- 250g fettuccine pasta (or gluten-free pasta of choice)
- 1 cup raw cashews, soaked in water for at least 2 hours
- 2 cups chicken broth
- 4 cloves garlic, minced
- 1 tablespoon nutritional yeast (optional)
- 1/2 cup unsweetened almond milk (or any non-dairy milk)
- 2 tablespoons olive oil
- Salt and pepper, to taste
- Chopped fresh parsley, for garnish

Instructions:

1. Drain the soaked cashews and rinse them thoroughly. In a blender, combine the cashews, chicken broth, minced garlic, nutritional yeast (if using), and almond milk. Blend until smooth and creamy. Set aside.

2. Bring a large pot of salted water to a boil. Cook the fettuccine according to package instructions until al dente. Drain and set aside.

3. In a large skillet, heat 1 tablespoon of olive oil over medium-high heat. Season the chicken strips with salt and pepper. Cook the chicken for about 5-6 minutes, or until cooked through and lightly browned. Take out the chicken from the skillet and set aside.

4. In the same skillet, add the remaining 1 tablespoon of olive oil. Pour in the cashew cream sauce and cook over medium heat, stirring constantly, until the sauce thickens slightly, about 3-5 minutes.

5. Add the cooked fettuccine and cooked chicken strips to the skillet with the cashew cream sauce. Toss everything together until well coated and heated through.

6. Divide the chicken Alfredo into serving plates. Garnish with chopped fresh parsley and additional black pepper, if desired.

Nutritional Information (per serving):

- **Calories:** 480 kcal
- **Fat:** 22 g
- **Carbohydrates:** 38 g
- **Proteins:** 32 g

AIP Meatloaf with Egg Yolks (Stage 1: Egg Yolks)

Prep Time: 20 minutes | **Cook Time:** 1 hour | **Servings:** 6

Ingredients:

- 800g ground beef (preferably lean)
- 2 egg yolks
- 1 onion, finely diced
- 2 cloves garlic, minced
- 1/2 cup chopped fresh parsley
- 1/4 cup coconut flour
- 1/4 cup unsweetened applesauce
- 2 tablespoons coconut aminos
- 1 teaspoon dried thyme
- 1 teaspoon dried oregano
- Salt and pepper, to taste

Instructions:

1. Preheat your oven to 350°F (175°C). Grease a loaf pan or line it with parchment paper.

2. In a large bowl, mix together the ground beef, egg yolks, finely diced onion, minced garlic, chopped parsley, coconut flour, unsweetened applesauce, coconut aminos, dried thyme, dried oregano, salt, and pepper. Mix until well combined.

3. Transfer the meat mixture into the prepared loaf pan, pressing it down evenly with a spatula or your hands.

4. Place the meatloaf in the preheated oven and bake for 50-60 minutes, or until the internal temperature reaches 160°F (71°C).

5. Take out the meatloaf from the oven and let it rest in the loaf pan for 10 minutes before slicing.

6. Slice the meatloaf and serve hot. Optionally, garnish with additional chopped parsley before serving.

Nutritional Information (per serving):

- **Calories:** 380 kcal
- **Fat:** 22 g
- **Carbohydrates:** 10 g
- **Proteins:** 34 g

Lamb Chops with Mint and Pomegranate Salad (Stage 2: Pomegranate Seeds)

Prep Time: 15 minutes | **Cook Time:** 10 minutes | **Servings:** 4

Ingredients:

- 8 lamb chops
- 1 cup fresh mint leaves, chopped
- 1/2 cup pomegranate seeds
- 1/4 cup extra virgin olive oil
- 2 tablespoons lemon juice
- 2 cloves garlic, minced
- Salt and pepper, to taste

Instructions:

1. Season the lamb chops with salt and pepper on both sides.
2. Heat a grill pan or skillet over medium-high heat. Cook the lamb chops for about 4-5 minutes per side for medium-rare, or adjust cooking time according to your preference and the thickness of the chops.
3. In a bowl, combine the chopped mint leaves, pomegranate seeds, extra virgin olive oil, lemon juice, minced garlic, salt, and pepper. Mix adequately to combine.
4. Arrange the cooked lamb chops on a serving platter. Spoon the mint and pomegranate salad over the lamb chops or serve it on the side.
5. Serve immediately while the lamb chops are hot and the salad is fresh.

Nutritional Information (per serving):

- **Calories:** 420 kcal
- **Fat:** 30 g
- **Carbohydrates:** 5 g
- **Proteins:** 32 g

Stuffed Bell Peppers with Ground Beef and Vegetables (Stage 3: Bell Peppers)

Prep Time: 30 minutes | **Cook Time:** 45 minutes | **Servings:** 4

Ingredients:

- 4 large bell peppers (any color), tops cut off and seeds removed
- 500g ground beef (preferably lean)
- 1 onion, finely chopped
- 2 cloves garlic, minced
- 1 zucchini, diced
- 1 carrot, diced
- 1/2 cup cauliflower rice
- 1 teaspoon dried oregano
- 1 teaspoon dried basil
- Salt and pepper, to taste
- 1 cup tomato sauce
- 1/2 cup beef broth
- Fresh parsley, chopped, for garnish

Instructions:

1. Preheat your oven to 350°F (175°C). Grease a baking dish large enough to hold the bell peppers upright.

2. Cut off the tops of the bell peppers and take out the seeds and membranes. If needed, trim the bottoms slightly to help them stand upright in the baking dish.

3. In a large skillet, brown the ground beef over medium-high heat until no longer pink. Drain excess fat if necessary. Add the chopped onion, minced garlic, diced zucchini, diced carrot, cauliflower rice, dried oregano, dried basil, salt, and pepper. Cook for 5-7 minutes, or until the vegetables are tender.

4. Spoon the ground beef and vegetable mixture into the hollowed-out bell peppers, pressing gently to pack the filling.

5. In a small bowl, mix together the tomato sauce and beef broth. Pour the mixture into the bottom of the baking dish around the stuffed peppers. Cover the dish with foil.

6. Bake in the preheated oven for 30-35 minutes, or until the peppers are tender.

7. Take out the foil from the baking dish. Sprinkle the stuffed peppers with chopped fresh parsley before serving.

Nutritional Information (per serving):

- **Calories:** 380 kcal
- **Fat:** 20 g
- **Carbohydrates:** 18 g
- **Proteins:** 32 g

Baked Cod with Almond Crust (Stage 2: Almonds)

Prep Time: 15 minutes | **Cook Time:** 20 minutes | **Servings:** 4

Ingredients:

- 4 cod fillets (about 150g each), skinless
- 1 cup almond flour
- 1/4 cup finely chopped almonds
- 1 teaspoon paprika
- 1/2 teaspoon garlic powder
- 1/2 teaspoon onion powder
- 1/2 teaspoon dried thyme
- Salt and pepper, to taste
- 2 eggs, beaten
- Lemon wedges, for serving

Instructions:

1. Preheat your oven to 400°F (200°C). Line a baking sheet with parchment paper.

2. In a shallow dish, combine the almond flour, chopped almonds, paprika, garlic powder, onion powder, dried thyme, salt, and pepper.

3. Pat the cod fillets dry with paper towels. Dip each fillet into the beaten eggs, then press into the almond mixture to coat evenly on both sides. Place the coated fillets on the prepared baking sheet.

4. Bake the cod fillets in the preheated oven for 15-20 minutes, or until the fish flakes easily with a fork and the crust is golden brown.

5. Remove from the oven and serve hot, garnished with lemon wedges.

Nutritional Information (per serving):

- **Calories:** 350 kcal
- **Fat:** 20 g
- **Carbohydrates:** 8 g
- **Proteins:** 32 g

Ginger-Turmeric Chicken Thighs with Tomato Relish (Stage 3: Tomatoes)

Prep Time: 15 minutes | **Cook Time:** 25 minutes | **Servings:** 4

Ingredients:

For the Chicken Thighs:

- 4 bone-in, skin-on chicken thighs
- 1 tablespoon olive oil
- 1 tablespoon grated fresh ginger
- 1 tablespoon grated fresh turmeric (or 1 teaspoon dried turmeric)
- Salt and pepper, to taste

For the Tomato Relish:

- 2 cups cherry tomatoes, halved
- 1/4 cup finely chopped red onion
- 2 tablespoons chopped fresh parsley
- 1 tablespoon extra virgin olive oil
- 1 tablespoon balsamic vinegar
- Salt and pepper, to taste

Instructions:

1. Preheat your oven to 400°F (200°C).

2. In a small bowl, mix together the olive oil, grated ginger, grated turmeric, salt, and pepper. Rub this mixture evenly over the chicken thighs.

3. Place the chicken thighs skin-side up on a baking sheet lined with parchment paper. Roast in the preheated oven for 20-25 minutes, or until the chicken is cooked through and the skin is crispy.

4. While the chicken is roasting, prepare the tomato relish. In a bowl, combine the halved cherry tomatoes, chopped red onion, chopped parsley, extra virgin olive oil, balsamic vinegar, salt, and pepper. Mix adequately to combine.

5. Serve the roasted chicken thighs hot, topped with the tomato relish.

Nutritional Information (per serving):

- **Calories:** 380 kcal
- **Fat:** 24 g
- **Carbohydrates:** 10 g
- **Proteins:** 30 g

Snacks Recipes

Deviled Eggs with Avocado (Stage 1: Whole Eggs)

Prep Time: 20 minutes | **Cook Time:** 10 minutes | **Servings:** 4

Ingredients:

- 4 large eggs
- 1 ripe avocado
- 1 tablespoon olive oil
- 1 tablespoon lemon juice
- Salt and pepper, to taste
- Paprika, for garnish
- Chopped chives, for garnish

Instructions:

1. Place the eggs in a saucepan and cover with water. Bring to a boil over medium-high heat. Once boiling, cover and remove from heat. Let sit for 10 minutes. Drain and cool the eggs under cold running water. Peel and halve lengthwise.

2. Scoop out the avocado flesh into a bowl and mash until smooth. Add olive oil, lemon juice, salt, and pepper. Mix adequately until combined.

3. Gently take out the yolks from the egg halves and add them to the avocado mixture. Mash together until smooth and creamy.

4. Spoon or pipe the avocado mixture evenly into the egg white halves.

5. Sprinkle paprika and chopped chives over the filled eggs.

6. Arrange on a serving platter and serve chilled.

Nutritional Information (per serving):

- **Calories:** 120 kcal
- **Fat:** 9g
- **Carbs:** 5g
- **Proteins:** 6g

Apple Slices with Almond Butter (Stage 2: Almonds)

Prep Time: 10 minutes | **Cook Time:** 0 minutes | **Servings:** 2

Ingredients:

- 1 medium apple, cored and sliced
- 4 tablespoons almond butter
- Optional toppings: sliced almonds, cinnamon

Instructions:

1. Core the apple and slice it into thin rounds or wedges.
2. Arrange the apple slices on a plate.
3. Place almond butter in a small bowl for dipping or drizzling over the apple slices.
4. Sprinkle sliced almonds and a dash of cinnamon over the almond butter, if desired.
5. Serve the apple slices with almond butter immediately.

Nutritional Information (per serving):

- **Calories:** 250 kcal
- **Fat:** 18g
- **Carbs:** 20g
- **Proteins:** 7g

Chia Seed Pudding with Coconut Milk and Honey (Stage 2: Chia Seeds)

Prep Time: 5 minutes | **Cook Time:** 0 minutes | **Chill Time:** 4 hours | **Servings:** 2

Ingredients:

- 1/4 cup chia seeds
- 1 cup coconut milk
- 1 tablespoon honey (optional, adjust to taste)
- Fresh berries, for garnish

Instructions:

1. In a bowl, combine chia seeds, coconut milk, and honey. Stir adequately until all ingredients are evenly mixed.

2. Cover the bowl and refrigerate for at least 4 hours or overnight. Stir once or twice during the first hour to prevent clumping.

3. After chilling, the chia seeds will absorb the liquid and thicken to a pudding-like consistency.

4. Stir the pudding before serving to redistribute the chia seeds.

5. Divide into serving bowls or jars.

6. Top with fresh berries or your choice of toppings, if desired.

7. Serve chilled and enjoy!

Nutritional Information (per serving):

- **Calories:** 250 kcal
- **Fat:** 20g
- **Carbs:** 15g
- **Proteins:** 5g

Celery Sticks with Sunflower Seed Butter (Stage 2: Sunflower Seeds)

Prep Time: 10 minutes | **Cook Time:** 0 minutes | **Servings:** 2

Ingredients:

- 4 celery stalks, trimmed and cut into sticks
- 4 tablespoons sunflower seed butter
- Optional toppings: sunflower seeds, sea salt

Instructions:

1. Trim the ends of the celery stalks and cut them into sticks of desired length.
2. Place sunflower seed butter in a small bowl for dipping or spreading onto the celery sticks.
3. Sprinkle sunflower seeds and a pinch of sea salt over the sunflower seed butter, if desired.
4. Arrange the celery sticks on a plate with the sunflower seed butter and toppings.

Nutritional Information (per serving):

- **Calories:** 180 kcal
- **Fat:** 14g
- **Carbs:** 10g
- **Proteins:** 6g

Trail Mix with Nuts and Dried Fruit (Stage 2: Mixed Nuts)

Prep Time: 5 minutes | **Cook Time:** 0 minutes | **Servings:** 4

Ingredients:

- 1/2 cup mixed nuts (such as almonds, walnuts, and cashews)
- 1/2 cup dried fruit (such as cranberries, raisins, or apricots)
- 2 tablespoons pumpkin seeds
- 2 tablespoons sunflower seeds
- Optional: 1/4 teaspoon sea salt (adjust to taste)

Instructions:

1. If the nuts are whole, chop them into smaller pieces if desired.
2. In a bowl, combine the mixed nuts, dried fruit, pumpkin seeds, and sunflower seeds. Add sea salt if desired and mix adequately.
3. Serve immediately, or store in an airtight container for later use.

Nutritional Information (per serving):

- **Calories:** 220 kcal
- **Fat:** 15g
- **Carbs:** 20g
- **Proteins:** 5g

<u>Baked Plantain Chips with Guacamole (Stage 3: Nightshade-free)</u>

Prep Time: 15 minutes | **Cook Time:** 20 minutes | **Servings:** 4

Ingredients:

For Baked Plantain Chips:

- 2 large green plantains
- 1 tablespoon olive oil
- Sea salt, to taste

For Guacamole:

- 2 ripe avocados
- 1 tablespoon lime juice
- 1/4 cup diced red onion
- 1/4 cup chopped cilantro
- Salt and pepper, to taste

Instructions:

1. Preheat the oven to 375°F (190°C).

2. Peel the plantains and slice them thinly using a mandoline slicer or a sharp knife.

3. Toss the plantain slices with olive oil until evenly coated. Arrange them in a single layer on a baking sheet lined with parchment paper.

4. Bake for 15-20 minutes, flipping halfway through, until the plantain chips are crisp and golden. Sprinkle with sea salt while still warm.

5. While the plantain chips are baking, prepare the guacamole.

6. In a bowl, mash the avocados with a fork until smooth or chunky, depending on your preference.

7. Add lime juice, diced red onion, chopped cilantro, salt, and pepper. Mix adequately to combine.

8. Serve the baked plantain chips with the guacamole on the side for dipping.

Nutritional Information (per serving):

- **Calories:** 260 kcal
- **Fat:** 18g
- **Carbs:** 26g
- **Proteins:** 3g

AIP Energy Balls with Flaxseeds (Stage 2: Flax Seeds)

Prep Time: 15 minutes | **Cook Time:** 0 minutes | **Chill Time:** 30 minutes | **Servings:** 12 balls

Ingredients:

- 1 cup unsweetened shredded coconut
- 1/2 cup ground flaxseeds
- 1/4 cup coconut oil, melted
- 1/4 cup raw honey or maple syrup (adjust to taste)
- 1 teaspoon vanilla extract
- Pinch of sea salt

Instructions:

1. In a mixing bowl, combine shredded coconut, ground flaxseeds, melted coconut oil, raw honey or maple syrup, vanilla extract, and a pinch of sea salt. Mix adequately until thoroughly combined.

2. Using clean hands, roll the mixture into 12 evenly-sized balls, about 1 inch in diameter.

3. Place the energy balls on a plate or tray lined with parchment paper. Chill in the refrigerator for at least 30 minutes to firm up.

4. Once chilled, serve the energy balls immediately, or store in an airtight container in the refrigerator for up to one week.

Nutritional Information (per ball):

- **Calories:** 120 kcal
- **Fat:** 9g
- **Carbs:** 8g
- **Proteins:** 2g

<u>Homemade Granola Bars with Pumpkin Seeds (Stage 2: Pumpkin Seeds)</u>

Prep Time: 15 minutes | **Cook Time:** 20 minutes | **Chill Time:** 1 hour | **Servings:** 12 bars

Ingredients:

- 1 1/2 cups rolled oats
- 1/2 cup pumpkin seeds
- 1/2 cup unsweetened shredded coconut
- 1/4 cup honey or maple syrup
- 1/4 cup coconut oil, melted
- 1/2 teaspoon vanilla extract
- 1/4 teaspoon sea salt
- 1/2 cup dried cranberries or raisins (optional)

Instructions:

1. Preheat your oven to 350°F (175°C). Line a baking dish or pan with parchment paper.

2. In a large bowl, combine rolled oats, pumpkin seeds, shredded coconut, and sea salt. Mix adequately.

3. In a separate bowl, whisk together honey or maple syrup, melted coconut oil, and vanilla extract until smooth.

4. Pour the wet ingredients over the dry ingredients. Stir until everything is evenly coated.

5. Transfer the mixture into the prepared baking dish or pan. Use a spatula or your hands to press it firmly and evenly into the pan.

6. Bake in the preheated oven for 20-25 minutes, or until the edges are golden brown.

7. Remove from the oven and let cool completely in the pan on a wire rack. Once cooled, refrigerate for at least 1 hour to firm up.

8. Lift the cooled granola slab out of the pan using the parchment paper overhang. Cut into 12 bars of equal size.

9. Serve immediately, or store the granola bars in an airtight container in the refrigerator for up to one week.

Nutritional Information (per bar):

- **Calories:** 180 kcal
- **Fat:** 10g
- **Carbs:** 20g
- **Proteins:** 4g

Mixed Berry Smoothie with Almond Milk (Stage 2: Almond Milk)

Prep Time: 5 minutes | **Cook Time:** 0 minutes | **Servings:** 2

Ingredients:

- 1 cup mixed berries (such as strawberries, blueberries, raspberries)
- 1 banana, sliced
- 1 cup unsweetened almond milk
- 1 tablespoon chia seeds
- Optional: 1 tablespoon honey or maple syrup (adjust to taste)
- Ice cubes (optional)

Instructions:

1. If using fresh berries, wash them thoroughly. Slice the banana.
2. In a blender, combine mixed berries, sliced banana, almond milk, and chia seeds. Add honey or maple syrup if desired.
3. Optionally, add a few ice cubes for a colder smoothie.
4. Blend on high speed until the mixture is smooth and well combined. If needed, scrape down the sides and blend again.
5. Pour the smoothie into glasses and serve immediately.

Nutritional Information (per serving):

- **Calories:** 150 kcal
- **Fat:** 5g
- **Carbs:** 25g
- **Proteins:** 3g

Raw Veggies with Tahini Dip (Stage 2: Sesame Seeds)

Prep Time: 15 minutes | **Cook Time:** 0 minutes | **Servings:** 4

Ingredients:

For Raw Veggies:

- 2 carrots, peeled and cut into sticks
- 2 cucumbers, sliced
- 2 bell peppers (any color), sliced

For Tahini Dip:

- 1/2 cup tahini (sesame seed paste)
- 1/4 cup water
- 2 tablespoons lemon juice
- 1 clove garlic, minced
- Salt, to taste

Instructions:

1. Wash and peel the carrots. Cut them into sticks.
2. Wash and slice the cucumbers and bell peppers into sticks or slices.
3. In a small bowl, whisk together tahini, water, lemon juice, minced garlic, and salt until smooth and well combined. Adjust the consistency with more water if needed.
4. Arrange the raw veggies on a serving platter.
5. Serve the tahini dip alongside the raw veggies.

Nutritional Information (per serving):

- **Calories:** 200 kcal
- **Fat:** 15g
- **Carbs:** 15g
- **Proteins:** 5g

Coconut Macaroons with Egg Whites (Stage 1: Whole Eggs)

Prep Time: 15 minutes | **Cook Time:** 20 minutes | **Servings:** 12 macaroons

Ingredients:

- 3 cups unsweetened shredded coconut
- 4 large egg whites
- 1/2 cup honey or maple syrup
- 1 teaspoon vanilla extract
- Pinch of salt

Instructions:

1. Preheat your oven to 325°F (160°C). Line a baking sheet with parchment paper.

2. In a mixing bowl, combine the shredded coconut, egg whites, honey or maple syrup, vanilla extract, and a pinch of salt. Mix adequately until all ingredients are thoroughly combined.

3. Scoop about 2 tablespoons of the mixture and form into compact mounds using your hands. Place each macaroon onto the prepared baking sheet, evenly spaced.

4. Bake in the preheated oven for 18-20 minutes, or until the macaroons are golden brown on the edges.

5. Remove from the oven and let cool completely on the baking sheet.

6. Once cooled, serve the coconut macaroons immediately, or store in an airtight container at room temperature for up to one week.

Nutritional Information (per macaroon):

- **Calories:** 180 kcal
- **Fat:** 12g
- **Carbs:** 15g
- **Proteins:** 2g

Sliced Cucumbers with Smoked Salmon and Dill (Stage 1: Nightshade-free)

Prep Time: 15 minutes | **Cook Time:** 0 minutes | **Servings:** 2

Ingredients:

- 1 cucumber, thinly sliced
- 4 ounces smoked salmon, thinly sliced
- Fresh dill, for garnish

Instructions:

1. Wash the cucumber thoroughly. Slice it thinly using a sharp knife or a mandoline slicer.
2. Thinly slice the smoked salmon.
3. Arrange the cucumber slices on a serving plate.
4. Top each cucumber slice with a piece of smoked salmon.
5. Garnish with fresh dill leaves.
6. Serve immediately as an appetizer or light meal.

Nutritional Information (per serving):

- **Calories:** 150 kcal
- **Fat:** 8g
- **Carbs:** 4g
- **Proteins:** 15g

Chapter 8

Guidance on Reintroduction

Understanding the Reintroduction Phase

The reintroduction phase of the Autoimmune Protocol (AIP) diet is an essential step aimed at helping you identify specific food triggers for autoimmune symptoms. Following the strict elimination phase, where potential inflammatory foods are removed, the reintroduction phase enables you to test and identify the foods your body can tolerate methodically and those it cannot. This phase is crucial for customizing your diet, supporting long-term health, and preventing autoimmune flare-ups by avoiding known triggers.

Preparing for Reintroduction

Properly preparing for the reintroduction phase guarantees a seamless and successful process. Here are a few steps to prepare:

- **Record Baseline Health:** Maintain a comprehensive log of your health condition after the elimination phase that includes symptom levels, energy levels, digestion, and overall sense of well-being.
- **Choose a Calm Period:** Start reintroduction when you are calm and stable, as external factors can make it difficult to identify food reactions accurately.
- **Plan and Prioritize:** Determine which foods you miss the most or consider essential to reintroduce first. Having a list to ensure the process stays organized would be helpful.
- **Collect Supplies:** Make sure to have a good supply of the foods you intend to reintroduce, making sure they are of excellent quality and free from additives or processing.

Step-by-Step Reintroduction Process

The reintroduction process involves a meticulous approach of gradually reintroducing foods and closely observing how your body reacts. Here are the steps to follow for each food:

- **Pick a Food:** Choose a single food item to reintroduce.
- **Introduce Gradually:** For optimal results, start with a small portion of the selected food, like a teaspoon or a small bite, on the first day. Pay close attention to any immediate reactions. If there are no reactions, you can increase the portion to a serving size on the second day.
- **Monitor for Reactions:** Wait for three days without introducing any additional new foods. Pay close attention to any symptoms or changes in your health during this period.
- **Record Observations:** It's essential to maintain a comprehensive record of your reactions, noting any symptoms like digestive issues, joint pain, fatigue, skin changes, or mood alterations.
- **Evaluate:** If there are no adverse reactions, the food can be deemed suitable for your diet. If any symptoms occur, please note them and refrain from eating the food.

Tracking and Monitoring Reactions

Accurate tracking and monitoring are crucial for identifying safe and trigger foods. Here are a few suggestions:

- **Symptom Diary:** Keep a symptom diary to track your daily health status and note any changes that may occur after reintroducing foods.
- **Detail Reactions:** Provide detailed information about the symptoms you experienced, such as how severe they were, how long they lasted, and how soon they appeared after eating the food.
- **Compare Baselines:** Regularly compare your current symptoms to your baseline health documented at the end of the elimination phase.
- **Use Tools:** Use tracking apps or spreadsheets better to easily organize your observations and spot patterns.

Identifying Safe Foods and Trigger Foods

As you continue the reintroduction phase, you'll need to sort foods into safe and trigger groups.

- **Safe Foods:** Foods that are unlikely to cause any adverse reactions and can be safely incorporated into your regular diet.
- **Trigger Foods:** Foods that can lead to symptoms or flare-ups, indicating that it's best to avoid them for the sake of your health.

It is common to experience unique responses to certain foods, and as tolerance levels can vary over time, it may be necessary to retest them later.

Adjusting the Diet Post-Reintroduction

After completing the reintroduction phase, make adjustments to your diet according to your findings:

- **Incorporate Safe Foods**: Gradually incorporate various nutritious foods into your daily meals to promote a safe and balanced diet.
- **Eliminate Trigger Foods:** Remove trigger foods from your diet to prevent symptoms and promote autoimmune health.
- **Balanced Diet:** Focus on a balanced diet that incorporates a wide range of vegetables, fruits, proteins, and healthy fats.
- **Routine Evaluation:** Reassess your diet periodically, as sensitivities and tolerances can change over time. It might be a good idea to consider retesting certain foods to assess any potential changes in how your body reacts.

The reintroduction phase is a personalized journey that helps you better understand your body and make well-informed dietary decisions. By following this process diligently, you can tailor the AIP diet to meet your specific requirements and experience lasting health benefits.

Chapter 9

Frequently Asked Questions and Troubleshooting

Common Questions About the AIP Diet

1. *What is the AIP diet?* The Autoimmune Protocol (AIP) diet is a specialized diet that aims to manage autoimmune conditions by reducing inflammation. It prioritizes nutrient-dense, whole foods and removes potential dietary triggers that may lead to immune system reactions.

2. *How long should I stay in the elimination phase?* The elimination phase usually lasts 30 to 90 days, although the length may differ depending on individual requirements and how one responds to it. It is crucial to wait until you notice a significant reduction in symptoms before starting the reintroduction phase.

3. *Is it possible to adhere to the AIP diet while following a vegetarian or vegan lifestyle?* Although the AIP diet mainly revolves around animal proteins, it can be modified to suit a vegetarian or vegan lifestyle by emphasizing AIP-approved plant-based protein sources and ensuring adequate nutrient intake.

4. *Can the AIP diet contribute to weight loss?* Although weight loss is not the primary objective of the AIP diet, several people have reported losing weight by reducing inflammation and consuming nutrient-rich foods.

5. *Is it possible to dine out while following the AIP diet?* Eating out can be challenging when on the AIP diet, but it's not impossible. When searching for restaurants, it's important to find ones that provide customizable options. Additionally, make sure to communicate any dietary restrictions you may have clearly. Choose straightforward dishes with few ingredients and steer clear of sauces or dressings that might have ingredients that don't meet the requirements.

Resolving Common Problems

1. *I haven't noticed any improvement in my symptoms. What course of action should I take?*

- **Check Compliance:** Ensure you strictly follow the AIP guidelines to avoid inadvertently consuming non-compliant foods.
- **Examine Ingredients:** Thoroughly examine labels and ensure that all foods and supplements adhere to the AIP guidelines.
- **Consult a Professional:** It may be beneficial to seek guidance from a healthcare provider or nutritionist with expertise in autoimmune conditions. They can help you identify any potential issues and make the necessary adjustments.

2. *I am experiencing fatigue and a lack of energy. Is this normal?*

- **Adjust Nutrient Intake:** Ensure you get the right amount of calories and a well-rounded mix of proteins, fats, and carbohydrates.
- **Monitor Nutrient Deficiencies:** Look out for possible deficiencies in vitamins and minerals, like iron, vitamin D, and B vitamins.
- **Hydration:** Drink plenty of water throughout the day to stay hydrated and maintain energy levels.

3. ***I'm experiencing digestive issues. What can I do?***

- **Slow Introduction:** Gradually introduce new foods to allow your digestive system to adjust.
- **Probiotics and Fermented Foods:** Include probiotic-rich foods and supplements to promote gut health.
- **Digestive Enzymes:** Consider incorporating digestive enzymes into your daily diet to assist with the breakdown of foods.

4. ***I'm having trouble resisting food cravings. What is the best way to handle them?***

- **Healthy Alternatives:** Seek AIP-friendly substitutes for your go-to dishes to satisfy your cravings.
- **Balanced Meals:** Ensure your meals are well-balanced and nutrient-dense to help you stay full and satisfied.
- **Mindful Eating:** Employ mindful eating techniques to maintain focus on your objectives and prevent impulsive eating.

Adjusting the Diet for Personal Needs

1. Customizing Your Diet to Fit Your Lifestyle

- **Meal Prep:** Plan and prepare meals in advance to save time and ensure you have AIP-compliant foods readily available.
- **Simple Recipes:** Focus on simple recipes suitable for your busy schedule and culinary skills.

2. Modifying the Diet for Specific Health Conditions

- **Additional Restrictions:** For people with multiple food sensitivities or other health conditions, it may be necessary to make further adjustments to the AIP diet to eliminate additional triggers.
- **Consultation:** Collaborate with a healthcare professional to develop a personalized plan catering to your health needs and conditions.

3. Modifying the Diet for Family and Social Situations

- **Inclusive Meals:** Create AIP-compliant meals that can be enjoyed by the entire family, promoting sustainability and inclusivity.
- **Communication:** Clearly convey your dietary requirements to friends and family to get their support and understanding at social gatherings.

4. Long-term Sustainability

- **Flexible Approach:** After identifying your trigger foods, try adapting the AIP diet to include a wider variety of safe foods.
- **Lifestyle Integration:** Incorporate the principles of the AIP diet into your long-term lifestyle by focusing on whole, nutrient-dense foods and avoiding known triggers.

By providing solutions to common questions, troubleshooting issues, and tailoring the diet to your specific needs, you can effectively navigate the AIP diet and experience improved health and well-being.

Conclusion

As you start and continue your journey with *"The Autoimmune Protocol Diet Cookbook for Beginners,"* remember that the AIP diet serves as a pathway towards reconfiguring your immune system and regaining your health. By prioritizing nutrient-dense, anti-inflammatory foods and removing possible triggers, you have made substantial progress in managing your autoimmune condition and improving your overall well-being.

This cookbook provides a wide range of delicious, AIP-compliant recipes, practical shopping tips, and comprehensive guidelines to help you successfully navigate the elimination and reintroduction phases. The journey may prove challenging at times, but the benefits of experiencing less discomfort, having increased energy, and enjoying better health make it all worthwhile.

As you progress, it's important to stay attuned to your body and make any necessary adjustments along the way. Embrace the principles of the AIP diet as a long-term, sustainable lifestyle choice. Embrace and appreciate your progress, be patient, and remember that each step takes you closer to an autoimmune disease-free life.

Thank you for choosing *"The Autoimmune Protocol Diet Cookbook for Beginners"* as your companion on this journey. May it inspire, nourish, and support you in achieving lasting health and happiness.

Recipes Index

A

B

C

D

E

G